Managing Hypertension

McFarland Health Topics

Living with Multiple Chemical Sensitivity: Narratives of Coping. Gail McCormick. 2001

Graves' Disease: A Practical Guide. Elaine A. Moore with Lisa Moore. 2001

Autoimmune Diseases and Their Environmental Triggers. Elaine A. Moore. 2002

Hepatitis: Causes, Treatments and Resources. Elaine A. Moore. 2006

Arthritis: A Patient's Guide. Sharon E. Hohler. 2008

The Promise of Low Dose Naltrexone Therapy: Potential Benefits in Cancer, Autoimmune, Neurological and Infectious Disorders. Elaine A. Moore and Samantha Wilkinson. 2009

Living with HIV: A Patient's Guide. Mark Cichocki, RN. 2009

Understanding Multiple Chemical Sensitivity: Causes, Effects, Personal Experiences and Resources. Els Valkenburg. 2010

Type 2 Diabetes: Social and Scientific Origins, Medical Complications and Implications for Patients and Others. Andrew Kagan, M.D. 2010

The Amphetamine Debate: The Use of Adderall, Ritalin and Related Drugs for Behavior Modification, Neuroenhancement and Anti-Aging Purposes. Elaine A. Moore. 2011

CCSVI as the Cause of Multiple Sclerosis: The Science Behind the Controversial Theory. Marie A. Rhodes. 2011

Coping with Post-Traumatic Stress Disorder: A Guide for Families, 2d ed. Cheryl A. Roberts. 2011

Living with Insomnia: A Guide to Causes, Effects and Management, with Personal Accounts. Phyllis L. Brodsky and Allen Brodsky. 2011

Caregiver's Guide: Care for Yourself While You Care for Your Loved Ones. Sharon E. Hohler. 2012

You and Your Doctor: A Guide to a Healing Relationship, with Physicians' Insights. Tania Heller, M.D. 2012

Autogenic Training: A Mind-Body Approach to the Treatment of Chronic Pain Syndrome and Stress-Related Disorders, 2d ed. Micah R. Sadigh. 2012

Advances in Graves' Disease and Other Hyperthyroid Disorders. Elaine A. Moore with Lisa Marie Moore. 2013

Cancer, Autism and Their Epigenetic Roots. K. John Morrow, Jr. 2014

Living with Bipolar Disorder: A Handbook for Patients and Their Families. Karen R. Brock, M.D. 2014

Cannabis Extracts in Medicine: The Promise of Benefits in Seizure Disorders, Cancer and Other Conditions. Jeffrey Dach, M.D., Elaine A. Moore and Justin Kander. 2015

Managing Hypertension: Tools to Improve Health and Prevent Complications. Sandra A. Moulton. 2016

Mammography and Early Breast Cancer Detection: How Screening Saves Lives. Alan B. Hollingsworth, M.D. 2016

Central Sensitization and Sensitivity Syndromes: A Handbook for Coping. Amy Titani. Forthcoming

Managing Hypertension

Tools to Improve Health and Prevent Complications

SANDRA A. MOULTON

MCFARLAND HEALTH TOPICS
Series Editor Elaine A. Moore

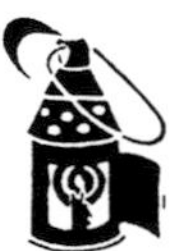

McFarland & Company, Inc., Publishers
Jefferson, North Carolina

Library of Congress Cataloguing-in-Publication Data

Names: Moulton, Sandra A., author.
Title: Managing hypertension : tools to improve health and prevent complications / Sandra A. Moulton.
Description: Jefferson, North Carolina : McFarland & Company, Inc., Publishers, 2016. | Series: McFarland health topics | Includes bibliographical references and index.
Identifiers: LCCN 2016039550 | ISBN 9780786494217 (softcover : acid free paper) ♾
Subjects: LCSH: Hypertension—Treatment. | Hypertension—Prevention.
Classification: LCC RC685.H8 M594 2016 | DDC 616.1/32—dc23
LC record available at https://lccn.loc.gov/2016039550

British Library cataloguing data are available

ISBN (print) 978-0-7864-9421-7
ISBN (ebook) 978-1-4766-2247-7

Printed in the United States of America

McFarland & Company, Inc., Publishers
Box 611, Jefferson, North Carolina 28640
www.mcfarlandpub.com

In memory
of my beloved mother, Louise,
who taught me the importance
of an education

Acknowledgments

I would like to thank God for giving me the health and strength to write my first book.

Thank you to Cheryl Saramak, my excellent typist and friend. I could not have done this without you.

To all of the wonderful contributors who made this book look great: thanks so much!

Thank you to Donald for helping me to stay focused and encouraging me to continue writing.

Thanks to my son, Christopher. Thanks to my family. Thanks also to my late friend, Janice Jackson, and friends Maureen Thorpe, Natalie, Dave, and Akin Falode. Thank you to my first cousin, Dominique Diedrick, for the excellent illustrations. Words cannot express my sincere gratitude for the support and kind words of encouragement from all of you.

Many thanks.

Table of Contents

Acknowledgments vi

Preface 1

Introduction 3

Part I

1. Hypertension: An Overview 7

Overview of Blood Pressure and High Blood Pressure 8
Are There Symptoms of High Blood Pressure? 8
Blood Pressure Measurements 9
Proper Steps to Measure Blood Pressure Manually 9
What Is Hypertension or High Blood Pressure? 11
Prehypertension 13
Risk Factors for Prehypertension 15
Prehypertension Stages 15
I've Been Diagnosed with Prehypertension. What Is the Course of Action? 15
Dentistry and Hypertension 18
Home Blood Pressure Monitoring 19
Classifications of High Blood Pressure 19
Etiology (Causes) of Hypertension 20
Adult Blood Pressure Levels 20
Risk Factors for Hypertension 22

2. Hypertension Prevalence 23

Prevalence of Hypertension in African Americans 23
Diseases Attributable to Hypertension 24
Statistics of Hypertension, Mortality, and Morbidity—A Brief Overview 27
Manifestation of Hypertension (Pathophysiology) 29
Sodium Sensitivity 29
Genetics 30
Natural History of Essential Hypertension 31
How Complicated Hypertension Affects Target Organs 31

Variation in Rates of High Blood Pressure by Age, Gender, and Race 33
Brief Overview: Role of the Heart in Blood Pressure 34
Position of the Heart 35

3. Cardiovascular Disease 36
Home Blood Pressure Monitoring 38
Negative Outcomes of Clinic Visits Versus Home Blood Pressure Monitoring 39
Self-Management for Hypertension Using Home Blood Pressure Monitoring 40
Ambulatory Blood Pressure Monitoring 44
Reducing Risk Factors of Coronary Heart Disease in Special Populations to Meet Healthy People 2020 Objective 47
Hypertension and Its Relation to Left Ventricular Hypertrophy 49
Prevalence of Cardiovascular Disease (CVD) 51
Definition of Heart Failure 53
Stages of Heart Failure 54
Heart Failure in Ethnic Minority Populations in Canada 55
Role of Diabetes and Coronary Artery Disease 56
Hypertension and Heart Disease in Diabetes 57
Some Coronary Artery Changes in People with Diabetes and Whether Vitamin D Deficiency Plays a Role 58
Biochemical Changes in Diabetes 61
Diabetic Atherosclerosis 61
Diabetic Coronary Plaque 61
Heart Disease Risk Factors 62

4. Vitamin D 64
What Is Vitamin D and How Is It Metabolized? 64
Functions of Vitamin D 65
Does Vitamin D Play a Role in the Development of Hypertension? 66
Some Food Sources of Vitamin D 68
The Connection Between Vitamin D Insufficiency and Blood Pressure: A Comparison 68
Lower Vitamin D Levels and Mortality 69
Parathyroid Hormone and Vitamin D Levels 71
Low Vitamin D Levels and Cardiovascular Disease 72

5. Kidney Disease 73
Brief Description of the Kidneys 73
Functions of the Kidneys 73
Causes of Kidney Disease 74
The Kidneys: Fluid Balance, Electrolytes, and Waste Products 75
Renin and Blood Pressure 76
Economic Impact of Kidney Disease in the United States 76
Two Major Complications of Chronic Kidney Disease (CKD) 77
Chronic Kidney Disease and Its Prevalence 77

Prevalence of End-Stage Renal Disease 79
Kidney Disease and Hypertension 79
Does Weight Play a Role in the Development of Chronic Kidney Disease? 80
Left Ventricular Hypertrophy and Hypertensive Chronic Kidney Disease 83
Diabetic Kidney Disease and Blood Pressure 84
Definition of Chronic Kidney Disease 84
The Five Stages of Chronic Kidney Disease and Their Detection 85
Modalities for Kidney Failure—Brief Statistics 86
Hypertension and Kidney Disease 86
Uncontrolled Blood Pressure and Chronic Kidney Disease 87
Autoimmune Diseases and Chronic Kidney Disease 87
End-Stage Renal Disease Treatment in the United States 88
Peritoneal Dialysis and Hemodialysis 89
Vascular Access: A Brief History of the Pioneers 90
Three Types of Vascular Access 90
Arteriovenous Fistula 90
Advantages of Arteriovenous Fistula 92
Disadvantages 92
Maintenance of Arteriovenous Fistula 92
Live Kidney Donors and African Americans 94

6. Stroke and Cerebrovascular Disease 96
Stroke Mortality Reduction in the United States 97
Risk Factors for Stroke 97
Possible Cause of Stroke 98
How Does Stroke Happen? 98
Prevalence of Stroke 99
Avoidable Deaths Statistics from Stroke, Hypertension, and Heart Disease in the United States 99
Strategies to Avoid Stroke Deaths 100
Mortality: Stroke 101
Lifestyle Changes for Decreasing Stroke Risk 101
Stroke Types 103
Economic Impact of Stroke 105
High Blood Pressure and Ischemic Stroke 105
Genetic Variation and Intracerebral Hemorrhage 107
Disparities in Stroke Risks 107
Effects After Stroke 112

Part II

7. Nonpharmacological Management for Hypertension 116
Individual Lifestyle Modifications for Hypertension Management 117
The Roundtable Recommendation for Blood Pressure Management: The Lifestyle Approach 119

An Overview of the GenSalt Study 121
Adherence Interventions: Lifestyle Modifications, Medicine and Home Blood Pressure Monitoring 122
Intervention Approach: Blood Pressure Improvement in Primary Care for African Americans 124
Utilization of Community Settings for Lifestyle Interventions 124
Church Interventions to Promote Lifestyle Changes 127
Dietary Supplements for Hypertension 128
Physical Activity for Hypertension Management 129
Hypertension: Gait Slowing in Older Adults 132
Nutritional Intake and Physical Activity as Cardiovascular Risk Factors 135
Self-Efficacy and Self-Care Management for Hypertension 138
A Review of Patient-Tailored Self-Management for Blood Pressure 139
Definition of Self-Management 140
Self-Management for Blood Pressure Control 140
Tailored Interventions' Effectiveness: Self-Management Behaviors for Chronic Diseases 142

8. Pharmacological Management for Hypertension 145
Hypertension and Increased Age 147
Consistent Care Versus Standard Care for Blood Pressure Control Among African Americans and Whites 148
Medicine 148
Forms of Medication Used for Hypertension 149
Functions of Blood Pressure Medications 149
Some Popular Blood Pressure Medications 149
JNC 8 Guidelines 153
Resistant Hypertension 154
A Glance: Hypertension Management by Various Hypertension Societies 159
Differences in Medication Response in Non-Hispanic Whites and African Americans 161
Medication Adherence 161
Factors or Barriers to Medication Adherence for Hypertension in Different Cultural Groups 163
Factors That Affect Medication Adherence in African Americans with Hypertension 167

9. Hypertension Case Stories 171
The Story of an African American Woman 171
The Case of Jasper (J.M.) 172
Janice: A New Diagnosis of Hypertension and Kidney Failure 173
Donald's Story 174

10. Hypertension: Prevalence, Consequences and Lifestyle Modification Factors 177
Hypertension Prevalence in Football Players 177

Prehypertension and Hypertension: Physical Therapists' Involvement 178
High Blood Pressure in Blacks 180
Question: Self-Report Questionnaires for Antihypertensive Medication Adherence 182
Cardiovascular Disease 183
Cardiovascular Disease Risk Factors: Differences in Various Ethnicities in Canada 187
Women and Coronary Artery Disease 190
Blood Pressure and Cardiovascular Disease 191
Chronic Kidney Disease (CKD) 193
End-Stage Renal Disease: Psychosocial Impact and Knowledge Needs 194
Overview of Vitamin D, Hypertension and Cardiovascular Disease 199
Summary 203

Appendix 1. Sample Five-Day Meal Plan 205
Appendix 2. Test Your Knowledge of Hypertension 211
Bibliography 215
Index 229

Preface

Hypertension or high blood pressure is a chronic health condition common worldwide. It affects people of different age groups, different cultural backgrounds and different socioeconomic statuses. Alarmingly, this disease is widely documented by researchers to increase the risk of heart disease, kidney disease, and stroke. This is especially so if a patient's blood pressure is not effectively controlled and managed. Moreover, hypertension is believed to be one of the major risk factors for cardiovascular disease, and "cardiovascular diseases, including stroke, are the leading causes of death worldwide" (Chiu, Austin, Manuel, & Tu, 2010, p. 182).

Although individuals of all ethnicities may suffer from hypertension and its consequences, research frequently demonstrates that high blood pressure is more prevalent and is more challenging to control and manage in non-Hispanic black adults. The burden of the disease is also more pronounced in this group. It is important to note that hypertension not only affects individual patients but also has an impact on their families, friends, and communities, and increases costs to society.

Because hypertension is so widespread and the impact of the disease is so prevalent, I thought that a book about hypertension for the general public would increase awareness of the disease and help people suffering from this condition.

Through my work as a registered nurse and my personal experience with family members and friends with hypertension, I am aware that this chronic disease can pose a challenge to control and manage. And it can be even more challenging for individuals and their loved ones with limited support.

Managing Hypertension differs from other books because it is specific to the care and management of hypertension. It is geared for people in North America and worldwide, with some emphasis on the African American and aging populations. Numerous books have emphasized the prevalence, morbidity and mortality rates of hypertension in people of different cultural backgrounds, but this author was unable to locate a specific book that included the management of hypertension in African Americans and other ethnic groups.

It is my belief that if people have the tools to help manage their chronic health condition, their health outcome could be improved. In addition, population health could also be improved if morbidity (illness) and mortality (death) rates are decreased or prevented in people with high blood pressure.

Because hypertension is a chronic disease, a combination of medications and self-care behaviors may play a significant role in controlling blood pressure, decreasing the occurrence of hypertension-related illnesses and preventing premature deaths. Therefore, improving hypertension care is crucial for the individual and society. Control measures will improve the quality of life and overall health of the general population. While health initiatives caused significant strides in blood pressure control between 1988–1994 and 2007–2008 across age, race, and sex groups, hypertension control was lower among individuals 18–39 years old and individuals 60 years and older and in Hispanics (Egan et. al., 2010).

The information in this book is intended to educate people about hypertension, its risk factors, primary prevention measures, and how people can effectively control and manage this chronic disease. This information will not only inform people about the basis of hypertension but also its dangers and why it is crucial to control and manage it. The book consists of two parts and is divided into ten chapters.

Part I provides readers with information on the two major types and causes of hypertension and its role in heart disease, kidney disease, and cardiovascular disease. Also included is a brief overview of hemodialysis and peritoneal dialysis, because most people with kidney failure will require dialysis treatment modalities to survive. Illustrations and tables are included to enhance the reader's interest in and understanding of hypertension.

Part II focuses on treatment measures, such as medication and lifestyle management, to control and manage hypertension and to prevent hypertension consequences, such as heart disease, stroke, and kidney disease. Case studies and illustrations are also included in Part II.

My goal for this book is to provide people with the information they need to help control and manage hypertension and to improve their health outcomes in the twenty-first century and beyond. On a large scale, the successful management of hypertension could decrease illness and death rates globally.

Introduction

A person diagnosed with hypertension needs to be actively involved in his or her care for effective blood pressure control.

Hypertension, often referred to by its other name, high blood pressure, is a chronic health condition that affects people of different ages, different cultural backgrounds, and different genders all over the world. Because this condition is so widespread, it is a priority to effectively treat and manage it. This focus should extend beyond North America to target individuals worldwide. It is vital that this disease be effectively controlled to prevent or decrease illnesses and death rates that are due, in part, to untreated hypertension.

The prevalence of hypertension and awareness of it varies throughout the world, with the highest prevalence reported in Africa with a 46 percent prevalence for adults (World Health Organization, 2013) and the lowest rates in the Americas at 35 percent. In 2012 in the United States, about 17 percent of the approximately 70 million people with high blood pressure were reported to be unaware of their condition (CDC Data Brief 133, 2013; CDC High Blood Pressure Facts, 2015). As a result, the disease is often untreated.

In the United States alone, only about 52 percent of people with diagnosed hypertension have blood pressure that is under control (CDC High Blood Pressure Facts, 2015). The CDC also reports that in the United States, an additional one-third of the adult population has prehypertension, a condition in which blood pressure readings are higher than normal but not yet in the high blood pressure range.

Some people may discover they have the disease almost by accident, for example, after a physical examination for a new job or a blood pressure check at a health fair. If people are not aware they have hypertension, they are not treated. This may explain why hypertension is considered a silent killer (Li, Kuo, Hwang, & Hsu, 2012).

Although hypertension affects people of all races, substantial U.S. studies show that it is more prevalent in African Americans than in whites (Ferdinand, Pool, Weitzman, Purkayastha & Townsend, 2011). African Americans experience greater pressure-related end organ damage, earlier onset of the disease, and lower blood pressure control rates (Ferdinand et al., 2011). Consistent with the findings of Barksdale and Metiko (2010), black Americans develop the disease at an earlier age, tend to have a much higher blood pressure average, and tend to have more aggressive hypertension compared to hypertension in white Americans. It is important to note that global studies show that while the highest prevalence of hypertension is found in Africa, other countries such as Spain and Japan also show a high prevalence of hypertension (World Health Organization, 2013; Kearney et al, 2005) and the reasons for these ethnic differences are explored in this book.

Anyone can develop high blood pressure; it is not limited to a specific group of people or specific age group although its incidence rises with age. Whenever a person suffers from high blood pressure, he or she is at risk for developing other health conditions, such as heart disease and stroke, the leading causes of death in the United States (Centers for Disease Control and Prevention [CDC], 2015). Therefore, it is necessary that people diagnosed with hypertension who are being treated for it adhere to treatment regimens for effective blood pressure control. Similarly, people susceptible to hypertension need to be proactive and have their blood pressure checked regularly by a health-care practitioner. People also need to maintain a healthy lifestyle to decrease their risk of developing hypertension and its complications.

My desire to write this book stemmed from my commitment and passion to improve the lives of people suffering from hypertension. I believe that if people are provided with information about hypertension, they can lead a healthy life with high blood pressure.

The chief purpose of this book is to increase public awareness of hypertension by educating people about it, how to prevent it, and how to manage it.

Drastic management, ongoing research, and increased awareness are necessary in communities worldwide if the lives of hypertensive people are to be improved and death rates decreased. These measures are vital to decrease the burdens of hypertension. African Americans need to be especially vigilant because hypertension is documented to be more widespread in this cohort and effective control and management pose greater challenges.

The information in this book comes from extensive research, ranging from online medical journal articles and reviews, observational studies, the results of research and clinical trials, consensus, and books. I've reviewed relevant literature from a variety of databases, such as Cumulative Index to Nursing and Allied Health Literature (CINAHL), PUB MED, and MEDLINE

EBSCO. I searched from 2004 to 2016 to obtain updated research material about the topic published in English and include the 2014 updated JNC 8 hypertension guidelines.

This is an informative book to have in your possession, whether you keep it in your office, classroom, or clinic, or use it as a reference guide. I have made every effort to make this book as interesting, educational, and easy to read as possible. Throughout, I refer to either hypertension or high blood pressure interchangeably, reflecting the use of these terms in relevant studies.

The book consists of two parts divided into ten chapters. Part I provides the tools needed for individuals to keep informed about the latest findings in hypertension. In the chapters of Part I, readers will also find information about prehypertension and the two major types of hypertension, how the disease manifests itself in the body, and the etiology, or causes, of hypertension.

Part I also briefly covers diabetes and its role in hypertension and heart disease. The chapters of Part I list dietary and socioeconomic factors in relation to hypertension risk in different races. The function of vitamin D and its role in hypertension and cardiovascular disease is also covered. Illustrations and easy-to-read tables have been added, and readers will also acquire information about peritoneal dialysis and hemodialysis in Part I.

Part II focuses on treatment. The chapters comprising Part II outline both pharmacological and nonpharmacological management for hypertension to prevent or reduce heart disease, stroke and kidney disease. Lifestyle measures such as exercise, smoking restrictions and dietary modifications are also outlined. The importance of medication management and adherence is also covered.

Last but not least, readers will find case studies and illustrations in the chapters of Part II. Additional information is provided in the appendixes.

It is my hope that readers will benefit from the material covered in this book, increasing their awareness and understanding of hypertension. It is important to note that this book is not intended to resolve the complications that may result from hypertension. Instead, it serves as a guide to assist people in controlling and managing hypertension effectively, with the goal of improving their health outcomes in the twenty-first century and beyond and decreasing the prevalence, morbidity and mortality rates in the population. In addition to reading this book, people with hypertension should always seek medical advice regarding their health conditions.

Let us embrace knowledge about hypertension to improve the health of people with hypertension worldwide!

PART I

1

Hypertension: An Overview

Diagnosis, treatment, and control of hypertension is necessary for decreasing the prevalence as well as the morbidity and mortality rates of people afflicted by it. These measures are vital not only in North America but worldwide. The morbidity, mortality and the cost to society of hypertension are of grave concern and may explain why Madhur, Riaz, Dreisbach and Harrison (2014) considered this disease a public health challenge. "Hypertension is one of the most common diseases facing the American public today, with elevated blood pressure representing the number one attributable risk for death worldwide" (Dodani, 2011, p. 1). Being hypertensive increases a person's risk for stroke, heart attack, heart failure, and kidney disease (Dodani, 2011). Similarly, "untreated hypertension is associated with premature mortality and morbidity, including fatal and nonfatal stroke, myocardial infarction, coronary heart disease, renal damage, and vascular death" (Venkata et al., 2011, p. 801).

For instance, in 2006 in the United States, the Centers for Disease Control (CDC, 2012) reported that Americans visited their doctors 40 million times for high blood pressure treatment, and 66.2 percent of adults who visited their doctor in that year had their blood pressure checked. The CDC (2012) further maintained that 69.9 percent of U.S. adults with high blood pressure utilized medications to treat the disease, while about one in five (20.4 percent) with the condition were unaware they even suffered from the disease. Yet, almost half of two billion prescriptions filled yearly are not taken correctly (Cuffee et al., 2013).

The Centers for Disease Prevention and Control reports that about 70 million Americans have hypertension (CDC 2015). In an earlier report Chapman, Schwartz, Boerwinkie and Turner (2002) pointed out that of the people diagnosed with hypertension approximately 85 percent are between stage one and two, which is considered mild to moderate essential hypertension. But despite many classes of antihypertensive agents and mechanisms of action that are available, blood pressure is adequately controlled in only about 52 percent of the patients being treated (CDC 2015; Konerman et al., 2011). Nonadherence to treatment can be responsible for a patient's perceived lack of control, and the patient's health status can also have an impact on adherence. Medication adherence and lifestyle are believed to be crucial elements for therapeutic success for individuals with hypertension (Ma, Chen, You, Luo & Xing, 2011).

These statistics are alarming and suggest that even though hypertensive individuals sought treatment for their condition, their blood pressure levels were not adequately controlled. Uncontrolled, prolonged high blood pressure puts hypertensive people at risk for blood pressure-related consequences. Therefore, people with hypertension need to follow the treatment prescribed by their doctors and implement meaningful lifestyle behaviors. Decreasing salt intake, exercising regularly, consuming only a moderate amount of alcohol, decreasing weight, and implementing dietary approaches to stop hypertension such as the Dash Diet are recommended for all people with hypertension (Wexler et al., 2008).

It is important to have a basic understanding of blood pressure and how hypertension manifests itself in the body. For this reason, this chapter provides an overview of blood pressure, hypertension, pathophysiology, etiology, natural history of essential hypertension, age factors, race, ethnicity variation levels, and the role of the heart. The text refers to African Americans and blacks interchangeably, as well as hypertension and high blood pressure interchangeably.

Overview of Blood Pressure and High Blood Pressure

What Is Blood Pressure?

Blood pressure (BP) is the force of blood as it pushes against the walls of the arteries when the heart pumps blood throughout the body. Each time an individual heart beats, which is about 60 to 70 times a minute at rest, the blood is pumped outward in the arteries. Additionally, when the heart beats and pumps blood, blood pressure is at its highest level. This is called systolic pressure. Blood pressure falls when the heart is resting between beats. This is called the diastolic pressure (Bunker, 2014; Sentry Health Monitors, 2012).

Are There Symptoms of High Blood Pressure?

People may have no idea that they have high blood pressure because the disease does not cause any symptoms. This is why it is called a "silent killer"

(Wedro, 2013, p. 2). While most people with high blood pressure do not have any signs or symptoms, even if blood pressure readings reach dangerously high levels, rarely, a few people with even mild conditions of hypertension may have headaches, shortness of breath, eye changes, dizzy spells, or nosebleeds. These signs and symptoms are not specific and usually do not occur until high blood pressure has reached a severe or life-threatening stage.

Blood Pressure Measurements

Blood pressure readings are displayed in two numbers, and either number can be elevated. The systolic blood pressure is the top number and the diastolic blood pressure is the bottom number. For example, 120 (systolic) over 80 (diastolic) is written as 120/80 mm Hg (millimeters of mercury). A patient's blood pressure measurement is "usually taken at the upper arm over the brachial artery" (Wedro, 2013, p. 2). The systolic pressure is the measurement of pressure produced when the heart contracts (pumps) (Bunker, 2014; Wedro, 2013); the diastolic pressure is the pressure in the arteries during the filling and resting of the heart between heartbeats (Wedro, 2013).

Vascular auscultation is a method of measuring arterial blood pressure, using a sphygmomanometer. It is recommended that a person's initial blood pressure measurement be taken on both arms because the pressures may vary by 5 to 10 mm HG in the arm. Blood pressure depends on the cardiac cycle. This means systolic pressure can be high and diastolic low (Kavanagh, 1987).

Korotkoff's sound is the sound that is heard during blood pressure measurement and this should be recorded as the first, fourth, and fifth phases of sounds; for example, 120/80/74. The first phase of Korotkoff sound is a tapping sound as the cuff is deflated, which is the systolic blood pressure measurement. When the murmur sounds of the second phase change to a tapping sound again, this is the third phase. When the third phase tapping sounds become muffled, this is the start of the fourth phase, and the fifth phase is when there is no sound whatsoever. The diastolic pressure is believed to be between the fourth and fifth phases (Kavanagh, 1987). Kavanagh (1987) and Bunker (2014) have outlined the appropriate ways to take a person's blood pressure. These steps follow.

Proper Steps to Measure Blood Pressure Manually

1. The person must be comfortable and relaxed. A sitting position is best, and the individual should be rested.

2. Position the person's arm so that it rests on a table with the brachial artery situated approximately at heart level. This will ensure there is no drift in pressure of systolic and diastolic readings.
3. Use a properly sized blood pressure cuff or automated electronic device, snugly secured.
4. For blood pressure to be heard, the stethoscope should not touch the cuff or the person's clothing.
5. Ensure the stethoscope is placed properly over the person's brachial artery.
6. Inflate the cuff to approximately 30 mm HG, then slowly lower the cuff pressure (Kavanagh, 1987).
7. The individual should avoid drinking coffee or tea or any fluid that has caffeine 30 minutes before having his or her blood pressure taken (Bunker, 2014).
8. The individual should avoid talking while blood pressure is being taken (Bunker, 2014). Figure 1 shows how blood pressure is taken.

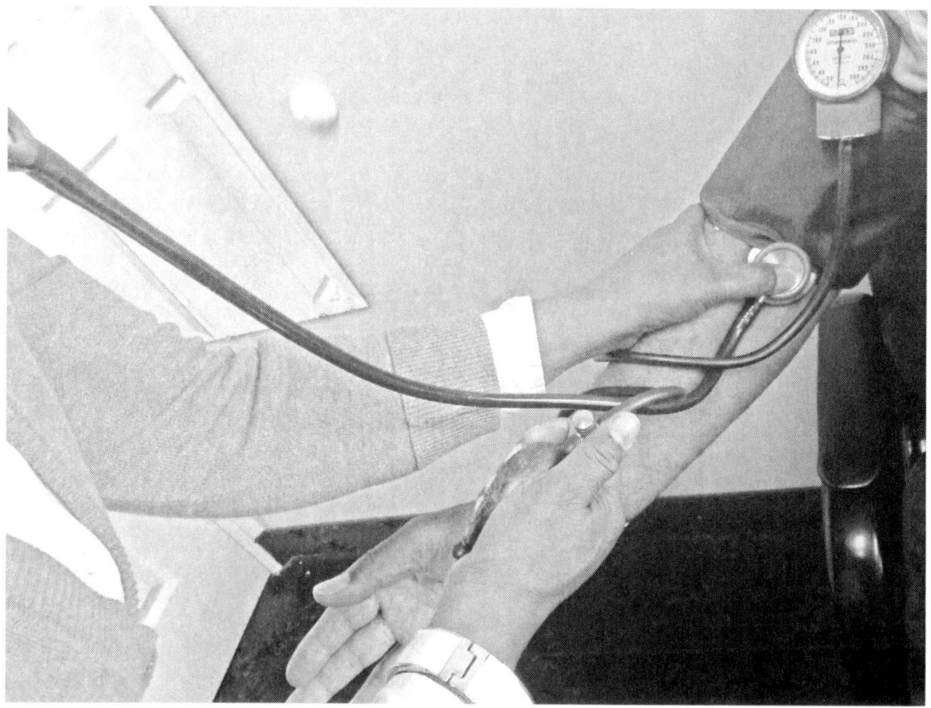

Figure 1. A dialysis patient has his blood pressure taken by a nurse. Blood pressure is not taken in an arm with an arteriovenous fistula.

In addition, recommendations from the 2014 Pharmacist's Letter/Prescriber's Letter include:

1. Measuring blood pressure after the patient has emptied their bladder and been seated for five minutes with back supported and legs resting on the ground but not crossed.
2. Taking two readings one to two minutes apart and averaging the readings (PL Detail Document. 2014).

What Is Hypertension or High Blood Pressure?

Hypertension is also called high blood pressure and "it is one of the most common worldwide diseases affecting humans" (Riaz et al., 2011, p. 1). Various medical groups have established definitions for hypertension and there is still controversy surrounding the recommendations, particularly those for patients older than 60 years. According to one of the most commonly used criteria in the United States, the Eighth Joint National Committee (JNC 8) guidelines, adults up to 60 years are classified as having hypertension if their systolic blood pressure is 140 mm Hg or higher, or diastolic blood pressure is 90 mm Hg or higher, or the patient is currently using antihypertensive medication (Hernandez-Villa, 2015). The JNC 8 guidelines were released in 2013 as an update to the JNC 7 guidelines, which were established in 2003. The two key changes in the newer guidelines versus JNC 7 are the less aggressive treatment guidelines for elderly patients and for patients younger than 60 years with diabetes and kidney disease, and withdrawal of the previous recommendation of only thiazide type diuretics as the initial therapy in most patients (Madhur and Maron, 2015).

The JNC 8 guidelines take specific situations into consideration. Based on the results of two Japanese studies, the VALISH and VATOS trials (Hernandez-Villa, 2015), the guidelines recommend not treating patients aged 60 years and older unless blood pressure is equal to or exceeds 150/90. A corollary recommendation is that patients whose systolic blood pressure is lower than the new guideline recommendation can continue current therapy if well tolerated.

In addition, the JNC 8 recommendations state that while a blood pressure of 140/90 is the target goal for patients ages 30–59 years, patients between 18 and 29 years may need treatment when blood pressure is lower on the basis of expert opinion. For patients aged 18 years or older with chronic kidney disease or diabetes, the guidelines recommend that treatment should be used to lower blood pressure to 140/90 bpm (Madhur and Maron, 2015). The JNC 8 guidelines also include recommendations for the type of pharmacological treatment used.

A scientific advisory issued in 2013 in collaboration with the American Heart Association, the American College of Cardiology, and the Centers for Disease Control and Prevention (CDC) also describes criteria for successful hypertension management including a blood pressure goal of 139/89 or less (Madhur and Maron, 2015).

The American Diabetes Association (ADA) released standard of medical care guidelines in 2011 that recommended nonpharmacological treatment for patients with mild hypertension (systolic BP 130–139 mm Hg or diastolic BP 80–89 mm Hg, which they report may be classified as prehypertension by other organizations.

The American Society of Hypertension (ASH) recommends a target BP of 140/90 for patients younger than 80 years of age, and a systolic BP of up to 150 mm Hg for patients 80 years and older. For patients 18 to 55 years of age, ASH recommends considering a lower target BP of 130/80 per prescriber discretion if treatment is tolerated. For patients with chronic kidney disease and an elevated albumin level (albuminuria) some experts recommend a target BP of 130/80 (PL-Detail Document, 2014).

In June 2013, the European Society of Hypertension and the European Society of Cardiology released new guidelines recommending that all patients should aim for a target systolic pressure of 140 or less with the exception of patients with diabetes and elderly whose recommendations should be based on their cardiovascular disease risk (Madhur and Maron, 2015).

The NIH's Systolic Blood Pressure Intervention Trial (SPRINT), which was conducted at 102 sites in the United States including Puerto Rico beginning in 2009, set out to show if a systolic BP of 120 mm Hg would further reduce the risk of kidney disease and other hypertension-related complications. The trial, which included 9361 participants ages 50 years and older, showed that among adults with hypertension but without diabetes, lowering systolic blood pressure to 120 mm Hg resulted in significantly lower rates of fatal and nonfatal cardiovascular events and death from any cause (SPRINT Research group, 2015). The NIH reports that they stopped the blood pressure intervention earlier than originally planned in an effort to quickly disseminate the significant preliminary results (National Institutes of Health 2015). The results of the SPRINT trial have led to many physicians adopting a target goal of 120 mm Hg for systolic blood pressure and generated controversy over the JNC 8 recommendations (Lunardo, 2016).

In light of the discrepancies between the various recommendations, Riaz et al. (2011) write that in clinical practice "a level for high blood pressure must be agreed upon for screening patients with hypertension and for instituting diagnostic evaluation and initiating therapy" (Riaz et al., 2011, p. 1). This may be necessary because some people may be prehypertensive before they develop full hypertension and patients with higher risk factors such as diabetics may require different therapeutic strategies.

The recommendations for target BP established by researchers in the United States are, in general, higher than those used globally. The World Health Organization defines normal blood pressure as a systolic BP of 120 mm Hg and a diastolic BP of 80 mm Hg (World Health Organization, 2013).

Prehypertension

According to the American Heart Association, prehypertension is a condition in which blood pressure consistently ranges 120–139/80–89 mm Hg. People with prehypertension are at risk for developing incident hypertension unless steps are taken to control it (*American Heart Association Heart and Stroke Encyclopedia*, 2016). In their report on the prevalence of hypertension, Egan and Stevens report that prehypertension affects 25–50 percent of adults worldwide and that the relative risk of incident cardiovascular disease (CVD) is greater with "stage 2" (130–139/85–89 mm Hg) than "stage 1" (120–129/80–84 mm Hg) prehypertension. In addition, their study found that relative risk of incident hypertension declines by approximately 20 percent with intensive lifestyle intervention, and by 34–66 percent with single antihypertensive medications (Egan and Stevens, 2015).

To assess the risk of coronary calcifications in prehypertension, the Coronary Artery Risk Development in Young Adults (CARDIA) study was carried out by Pletcher et al. (2014). The study cohort consisted of 3560 individuals, both black and white men and women, ages 18 to 30, from four cities in the United States.

This study used CARDIA's repeated blood pressure measures, started at the beginning of adulthood and continued over 20 years of follow-up. Pletcher et al. (2014) looked at individuals who were diagnosed with prehypertension between the ages of 20 and 35. The researchers evaluated whether a diagnosis of prehypertension before the age of 35 was associated with coronary calcium levels measured later in life.

The study found that coronary calcium later in life was strongly associated with young adults who showed signs of prehypertension before age 35. It was also shown that systolic prehypertension had a stronger association than diastolic prehypertension with coronary calcium. It is important to note that systolic prehypertension was common among black individuals, men, individuals of low socioeconomic status or of low education, and obese persons. Pletcher et al. (2014) emphasized the importance of targeting blood pressure control because prehypertension in black individuals occurred more in young adulthood. The authors also estimated a 70 percent higher probability of young prehypertensive individuals getting coronary calcium later in life than individuals with a systolic blood pressure that remained below 120 mm Hg until 35 years of age, regardless of an increase in blood pressure and other risk factors later in their lives.

The authors further stated that their findings provided a new basis for the relatively low blood pressure goal that was advocated by the Joint National Committee on Prevention, Detection, Evaluation and Treatment of High Blood Pressure (JNC 7). They stressed the need to address prehypertension with lifestyle changes, especially during young adulthood. The authors believe that their findings, which revealed that prehypertension in young adults is linked to coronary calcium later in life, is worth addressing.

The researchers supported their findings with other studies on middle-aged and older adults that linked prehypertension with cardiovascular disease, and studies on children or young adults that showed "cross-sectional association between blood pressure levels and atherosclerosis."

Pletcher et al. (2014) believe that optimizing blood pressure in young adults poses a great challenge. Pletcher and his colleagues pointed to a study of adults younger than 40 years old. The study showed that high blood pressure awareness was lower in younger individuals, that they were less likely to take medication even when made aware, and they were less likely to be adequately treated, compared to older people with hypertension.

The findings demonstrated the need for more stringent blood pressure screenings and control, especially in younger people. Healthcare practitioners are in the best position to fulfill this role. Implementing health promotion strategies in communities at an early stage is also vital. These strategies should be aimed toward at-risk individuals to educate and increase their awareness about prehypertension and its consequences. It is also necessary for physicians to carefully monitor people at risk for prehypertension. Physicians as well as policy makers should reinforce the need for lifestyle changes to help decrease an individual's chances of health problems, for instance, developing cardiovascular disease that could have been avoided by lifestyle changes to address prehypertension. Additionally, individuals need to be proactive, adjusting their lifestyles to ensure good health, because prehypertension blood pressure has been reported to be predictive of vascular disease mortality (Jorgensen & Maisto, 2008).

Government also plays a significant role in ensuring healthier communities and addressing socioeconomic disparities. If people can make better choices with the help of resources, they can lead healthier lives. The World Health Organization reports that interventions must be affordable, sustainable and effective and they do not recommend vertical programs that only focus on hypertension. Rather they advocate programs that address total cardiovascular risk. Globally, hypertension is responsible for at least 45 percent of deaths due to heart disease and 51 percent of deaths due to stroke (World Health Organization, 2013).

Risk Factors for Prehypertension

Risk factors for prehypertension include: being overweight or obese, which increases the amount of blood needed to supply oxygen and nutrients to tissues, which, in turn, increases the force on artery walls; age, with younger patients more likely to have prehypertension and older adults more likely to have hypertension; sex, with prehypertension more common in women through about age 45 years; race, with prehypertension particularly common among blacks; family history, especially if first-degree relatives are affected; sedentary lifestyle, which includes a risk of prehypertension as well as being overweight; diet high in sodium or low in potassium; tobacco use and secondhand smoke; alcohol when more than two drinks daily for men 65 years or younger are consumed or more than one drink a day for women of any age. For men older than 65 years, more than one drink daily can increase the risk for prehypertension; and other chronic conditions, including kidney disease, sleep apnea, and diabetes (Mayo Clinic, 2015).

Prehypertension Stages

There are different stages in the move from prehypertension to hypertension. These stages, which are highly variable, can occur in different age groups, with each stage having a different impact on body systems. The prehypertensive stage is mostly seen in people aged 10 to 30 years when there is increased cardiac output. It may then progress to early hypertension in people aged 20 to 40 years, with notable increased peripheral resistance. Finally established hypertension is more likely to be found in people aged 30 to 50 years, although the risk of established hypertension increases with age. Lastly, complicated hypertension is most likely to be seen in individuals aged 40 to 60 years (Riaz et al., 2011) and in people with co-existing conditions such as diabetes.

I've Been Diagnosed with Prehypertension. What Is the Course of Action?

Whenever people are told by their doctors that they have prehypertension, it means the blood pressure measurement is elevated above the normal reading but not high enough for the patient to be formally diagnosed with hypertension. However, having prehypertension is a relatively high risk for developing hypertension in the near future (Fogoros, 2011). If a person's blood pressure levels are higher than the normal range, his or her cardiovascular risk starts to increase. Thus, the higher the blood pressure, the higher the person's risk (Fogoros, 2011).

Although several randomized clinical trials have shown that aggressive treatment of hypertension can improve a person's outcome, trials for prehypertension are in the early stages of development and haven't proven that aggressive antihypertensive drug treatment causes better outcomes (Fogoros, 2011). Consistent with Pletcher et al. (2014), Fogoros (2011) believed that treatment of prehypertension with antihypertensive medications during young adulthood would be beneficial. Because there has been no randomized trial confirming the benefits in young adult populations, factors such as cost and potential side effects from long-term exposure to the medication would need to be looked at, given that there are no benefits against which to make a comparison (Pletcher et al., 2014).

Therefore, the recommended treatment for healthy prehypertensive individuals is to stop smoking and avoid excess alcohol intake (Fogoros, 2011). It is also recommended that to decrease the risk of developing hypertension from prehypertension, it is necessary for people to modify their lifestyle or behaviors. Dietary modification measures such as increasing potassium intake, decreasing fat and sodium intake (for example, Dietary Approach to Stop Hypertension [DASH]), increasing physical activity and maintaining a healthy weight can help some decrease their risk. But for others with certain health conditions, drug therapy is recommended. Fogoros (2011) states that clinical evidence revealed that more aggressive treatment improves outcomes. As a result, the author suggests drug therapy to help bring blood pressure levels to the normal range. This is recommended for people with conditions like coronary artery disease, peripheral artery disease, diabetes or chronic kidney disease. Fogoros (2011) further emphasizes that because prehypertensive people are at risk for getting actual hypertension, they should recheck their blood pressure at least every six to 12 months.

Jorgensen and Maisto (2008) pointed to the need to institute prevention measures for prehypertension especially in children, adolescents and college students because of its associated risk factor for people who develop primary hypertension in early adulthood. These measures are required to increase lifespan without the consequences of cardiovascular disease (CVD), which can result in morbidity and mortality at later stages of life. They believe the population to look at in the investigation of CVD risk and reductions is young adults who are enrolled in colleges and universities. Since it was reported many years ago that heavy alcohol intake is associated with high blood pressure, Jorgensen and Maisto (2008) believe it is a vital modifiable risk factor. The researchers further stated that a person's risk for having primary hypertension increases with three or more drinks per day.

In an effort to determine whether prehypertension and alcohol-related hypertension risk (ARHR) was predictive of primary hypertension (PH) among university undergraduate students, Jorgensen and Maisto (2008) conducted a study. The researchers used sex, parental history status, body mass index (BMI) and age for their study. Study participants consisted of 211 undergraduate women and men, aged 21 to 35 years, reported to be in good health, of which 95 were women.

The researchers found that a higher proportion of men were prehypertensive. Even though the men's risk for high blood pressure due to reported drinking was higher than the women's, the difference was not significant. But regardless of participants' BMI, age, sex, and their reported parental history of hypertension, "college students with prehypertension blood pressure levels were nearly four times more likely to report heavy drinking on a weekly basis" (Jorgensen & Maisto, p. 23). The findings also showed that prehypertension and heavy consumption of alcohol increases risk for primary hypertension.

The findings led the authors to emphasize the need for public health research studies in two areas: (1) carrying out tracking studies, and (2) studies to determine whether a reduction in alcohol intake "has salubrious effects on the cardiovascular system" (Jorgensen & Maisto, 2008, p. 24). They believed that the tracking study should be done during the undergraduate years and should look at "the effects of alcohol consumption on prehypertension and preclinical markers of CVD, such as arterial stiffness and left ventricular hypertrophy" (p. 24). The authors stated that it is vital to monitor prehypertension and also to assess the effectiveness of decreased alcohol consumption, because these measures will help to decrease blood pressure or prevent blood pressure from increasing during the college years.

Jorgensen and Maisto (2008) stated that because heavy consumption of alcohol is linked to hypertension, the implementation of effective interventions for heavy drinking might promote favorable effects in two of the health domains for college students: reduction in drinking-related injury and death, and reduction of cardiovascular disease later in life.

It would be worthwhile to adapt courses in university or college curriculums for young adults to include healthy lifestyle behaviors courses that would increase student awareness of alcohol and its impact not only on CVD but the entire body system. The various systems of the body work together to function, and a breakdown in one system may lead to imbalances. Further investigation should determine whether enrollment in university and coping with the university lifestyle or workload contribute to heavy consumption of alcohol.

Dentistry and Hypertension

The literature published on blood pressure has pointed to a prevalence of undiagnosed prehypertension and hypertension in dental patients. Dental appointments provide good opportunities to help identify prehypertension and hypertension and to increase individuals' awareness. Because white-coat hypertension can occur when BP is tested in a medical setting, abnormal readings should be investigated further by the patient's physician.

For instance, Al-Zahrani's (2011) study assessed the prevalence of hypertension and prehypertension in 208 female dental patients, ages 18 and over, who were being treated in KAUFD, a dental school treatment facility for only females in the western part of Saudi Arabia. Forty-two percent of the individuals were 41 years old and over. The researcher obtained individuals' sociodemographic information, hypertension history, medications used for hypertension, and systemic diseases as well as smoking history. Individuals' blood pressure measurements were taken twice by a dentist. JNC 7 criteria for blood pressure classification were used to determine which individuals were prehypertensive and hypertensive, and the average blood pressure measurement was used to analyze their findings. It is important to note that this study utilized the definition of prehypertension as blood pressure between 120/80 and 139/89 mm Hg. High blood pressure was considered a systolic blood pressure of 140 to 159 mm Hg or 90 to 99 diastolic (stage 1 hypertension), whereas stage 2 hypertension was individuals with a systolic blood pressure greater than 160 mm Hg or diastolic greater than 100 mm Hg.

The result of the study showed that 18 percent of the patients had elevated blood pressure, as well as 26 percent of those over 30 years old. It was also shown that in approximately half of the individuals with a history of hypertension, blood pressure was also elevated. It was revealed that more than half of the study individuals were either hypertensive or prehypertensive.

The researcher further stated that dentists need to assess the individual as a whole as part of a routine dental routine visit to ensure individuals' overall health, which can be done by appropriately screening, diagnosing, and referring patients. The author also believed that individuals would benefit from a referral to a primary care physician, given the high percentage of individuals who were hypertensive or prehypertensive.

According to Al-Zahrani (2011), a majority of dental patients who are at high risk for hypertension complications are probably not screened or evaluated in dental clinics. Al-Zahrani (2011) further stated that blood pressure measurement is not always a routine practice in dental clinics, even though it is recommended that all new dental patients should have their blood pressure taken. The finding suggests the need to increase dentists' awareness of prehypertension and hypertension to ensure that their patients are properly diagnosed and treated. Also if dental patients are made aware of their blood pressure condition, they may develop lifestyle changes to prevent hypertension consequences. Dental patients may also be affected by white-coat hypertension or white-coat syndrome, a condition in which blood pressure is elevated by anxiety when individuals are in the presence of physicians and other healthcare professionals. In this case, readings are elevated at office visits but remain normal when taken in the home setting. As much as 20 percent of the population are affected by white-coat syndrome (Sine, 2008).

Home Blood Pressure Monitoring

Home blood pressure monitoring is another method that can be useful in monitoring people with prehypertension. Monitoring blood pressure at home can serve to raise both the individual's and his or her doctor's awareness of changes in blood pressure levels. This method of monitoring can also prevent the misinterpretation of white coat hypertension. Therefore, if blood pressure is being monitored at home or the workplace at regular times every day, it will assist the practitioner in arriving at a diagnosis of prehypertension and hypertension.

Home blood pressure monitoring helps with the reporting of the person's true blood pressure, and this method will provide doctors with a log of blood pressure readings over time. In addition, Bosworth et al. (2011) report that home blood pressure measurement gives an indication of target organ damage and may decrease unneeded treatment of people with white coat hypertension.

Classifications of High Blood Pressure

There are two types of high blood pressure: (1) essential (primary), and (2) secondary. It is important to note the differences between these two types.

For example, there is no identified cause for essential high blood pressure (Riaz et al., 2011); its origins are not known (Jorgensen & Maisto, 2008). The causes of secondary high blood pressure such as kidney disease can be diagnosed (Riaz et al., 2011). Therefore, if high blood pressure develops over time and there is no cause for this development, it is considered essential hypertension. It is estimated that of the 70 million American adults with hypertension, 95 percent of those have essential hypertension, while fewer than 5 percent are reported to have secondary hypertension (Riaz et al., 2011).

Etiology (Causes) of Hypertension

Primary or essential hypertension usually has no clear cause although it may develop as a result of environmental (poor diet, lack of exercise, obesity) or genetic causes. Secondary hypertension may have several causes. Secondary hypertension which develops in response to another underlying condition includes renal, vascular and endocrinological causes (Riaz et al., 2011).

The causes of secondary hypertension are shown in Table 2 and the causes of primary hypertension in Table 3, which are found in Chapter Two.

Adult Blood Pressure Levels

High blood pressure has two levels. The categories of blood pressure levels in adults are outlined in Table 1.

Table 1.
Categories of Blood Pressure Levels in Adults

Category	*Systolic (top number) (mm HG)*	*Diastolic (bottom number) (mm HG)*
Normal	Less than 120	Less than 80
Prehypertension	120–139	80–89
Stage 1 HBP	140–159	90–99
Stage 2 HBP	160 or higher	100 or higher

Adapted from Sentry Health Monitors, http://www.lifeclinic.com/focus/blood/whatisit.asp, retrieved 06/03/2012, p. 1.

Aekplakorn et al. (2012) reported that their 2004 study showed that one of every five Thai people aged at least 15 years has high blood pressure. Moreover, "the proportions of awareness, treatment and control in hypertensive individuals are substantially below the target" (p. 1734).

Between 2004 and 2009, the Thai National Health Examination Survey

(NHES) looked at whether there were changes in the prevalence of hypertension and related awareness, treatment, and control of blood pressure and comorbidity in the general Thai population. The survey considered male and female adults in rural and urban areas. The age groups were 15 to 29, 30 to 44, 45 to 59, 60 to 69, 70 to 79, and greater than 80 years old. This study showed that the prevalence of hypertension was stable from 2004 to 2009 in this population. The authors pointed out that even though the prevalence rate was stable during this time period, it did not correspond with stable systolic blood pressure in this population. Most alarming was the lack of awareness and control of blood pressure in all age groups and both sexes, even with the improvements in awareness and control of the disease. For instance, half of the individuals knew they had hypertension, while only a quarter of the subjects had blood pressure that was controlled. But despite the findings indicating that detection and control of hypertension were low, Aekplakorn et al. (2012) observed that detection and control rates had improved in 2009.

They further stated that prehypertension prevalence decreased as individuals aged. This decline was noted to be greater in rural areas than urban areas. Additionally, as individuals aged, hypertension prevalence increased, and this increase was noted to be higher in urban areas than rural areas. In comparing males and females, hypertension awareness, treatment, and control levels were lower for males. Also, there was a significant difference between subjects with high BMIs, in that they had greater prevalence of high blood pressure. Additionally, rates of awareness, treatment, and control were lower in the rural settings (p. 1736), and this was found to be the case in both males and females. Furthermore, people less than 40 years of age "were less likely to be aware, treated and controlled when compared to others in older age groups" (p. 1740).

Patients were more likely to control their blood pressure if they were obese and had diabetes. Prehypertension and hypertension prevalence was also believed to be greater in individuals with lower levels of education.

The authors credited the general improvement in Thailand's quality of life in detecting hypertension. But they pointed to other studies that showed an increase in the prevalence of obesity in Thailand and the grave need for implementing strategies to manage and combat not only chronic communicable diseases but also hypertension and metabolic risk factors, with a great emphasis on obesity and hypercholesterolemia hypertensive subjects. The authors believe that the implication of their findings could further improve the quality of hypertension management and be beneficial for Thai policy planners and healthcare professionals.

Risk Factors for Hypertension

Researchers have identified multiple risk factors for developing hypertension. Many of these are controllable, while some are not. The following risk factors were identified by Wedro (2013):

Risk Factors That Cannot Be Controlled

- Age
- Race
- Socioeconomic status
- Family history and Genetic Influences
- Gender

Risk Factors That Can Be Controlled

- Obesity
- Sodium intake
- Use of alcohol
- Use of birth control pills
- Physical inactivity
- Medications

2

Hypertension Prevalence

According to the World Health Organization, in 2008, worldwide, approximately 40 percent of adults aged 25 and older had been diagnosed with hypertension. The number of people with the condition rose from 600 million in 1980 to 1 billion in 2008. The prevalence of hypertension is highest in the African Region at 46 percent of adults aged 25 years and older, while the lowest prevalence at 35 percent is found in the Americas. Overall, high-income countries have a lower prevalence of hypertension than low-income countries (World Health Organization 2013).

Prevalence of Hypertension in African Americans

The need to adequately control high blood pressure is significant, especially for African Americans. This is because hypertension is believed to be more prevalent in this group than it is in whites, yet it is less controlled, and the disease is linked to greater rates of cardiovascular disease, illness and death (Coly et al., 2008). For instance, the CDC high blood pressure facts (2012) reported on the burden of high blood pressure in the United States, stating that African Americans develop high blood pressure at an earlier age and that this group also develops the disease more often than whites and Mexican Americans. Barksdale and Metiko (2010) also found that black Americans develop the disease at an earlier age, their blood pressure average tends to be much higher, and their hypertension is more aggressive when compared to white Americans with the same disease.

Further, Nesbitt, Shojaee and Maa (2014) reported that hypertension is more prevalent in blacks in the United States, compared to other ethnic groups. The age-adjusted prevalence of hypertension is 40 percent in black adults compared to an overall prevalence of 29 percent for adults in the United States (CDC, 2015). The authors also confirmed that the severity of hypertension is greater, the onset is earlier, and the resulting cardiovascular disease rates are higher in this demographic compared to non–Hispanic whites.

Diseases Attributable to Hypertension

In terms of the diseases that are said to be attributed to hypertension, Nesbitt et al. (2014) reported that these consequences are higher in blacks than whites. For instance, nonfatal stroke rates in blacks are 1.3 times as high as in whites, fatal stroke 1.8 times, heart disease death 1.5 times, and end-stage kidney disease 4.2 times. Moreover, the death rates related to hypertension are staggering in African American persons compared to their white counterparts. According to Hicken, Lee, Morenoff, House and Williams (2014), deaths are about 15 per 100,000 people for white males and females, whereas in black females it is 40 per 100,000 and in black males greater than 50 per 100,000.

Other studies have also documented the prevalence of hypertension and predisposing health conditions to be greater in African American adults. For example, African Americans tend to experience greater pressure-related end organ damage, and their blood pressure control rates are lower compared to white Americans. The control rate is 23 percent for African Americans and 32 percent for white Americans (Ferdinand et al., 2011). In blacks, this disease is the main cause of cardiovascular illnesses and death, and these individuals are more likely to suffer from myocardial infarction, heart failure, and chronic kidney disease due to blood pressure that is not controlled. Moreover, the prevalence rate of hypertension in African American women residing in the United States is 45.7 percent, while it is 43.0 percent for African American men. Among their counterparts, the prevalence of hypertension is 33.9 percent in white men and in white women it is 31.3 percent (Cuffee et al., 2013).

These alarming statistics suggest a grave need for policy planners to conduct a systematic review and to implement strategies in communities to help control the prevalence of high blood pressure. These strategies may help to decrease the burdens of noncommunicable diseases, such as high blood pressure, in this population and improve the health outcomes of individuals.

This review is necessary because hypertension rates in the United States, despite showing improvement in recent years have remained high over the years. For instance, Go et al. (2014), in their 2014 Heart Disease and Stroke Statistics update from 2007 to 2010, showed that approximately 33 percent of adults in the United States over 20 years of age have high blood pressure. It is believed by Hicken et al. (2014) that racial and ethnic disparities in hypertension are responsible for some of the social disparities in health in the United

States, and they point to an estimated 40 percent prevalence of hypertension in black adults compared to 30 percent in white adults. Furthermore, the disparities are shown "in the larger burden of hypertension-related health and economic costs carried by non-white than white Americans (Hicken et al., 2014, p. 117).

But despite treatments, such as medication and behavioral therapies, there are still major gaps in controlling blood pressure. For example, as of 2012, more than half of the 70 million adults with this condition in the United States had uncontrolled blood pressure (Majid et al., 2012). According to Majid et al. (2012), whenever blood pressure is not controlled, the risks are greater for blood pressure–related consequences, such as stroke, acute myocardial infarction, kidney failure, and congestive heart failure.

Peralta, Katz, Newman, Psaty and Odden (2014) found that end-stage renal disease (ESRD), when compared to whites in the United States, is disproportionately higher in blacks and Hispanics. Not only is ESRD higher in blacks, but African Americans and lower socioeconomic individuals also "suffer a disproportionate burden of morbidity and mortality from cardiovascular disease" (Cooper et al., 2011, p. 1297).

Norris, Tareen, Martins and Vaziri (2008) also found that even though "the prevalence of chronic kidney disease (CKD) is similar across ethnic groups in the United States" (p. 538), ESRD is 1.5 to 4 times higher among minority groups, compared to whites, which indicates an increased difference in the progression of CKD.

Despite heightened awareness and the efforts to control hypertension in some hypertensive blacks, prevention and awareness of hypertension should be reinforced, and individuals and communities must play a key role in implementing these strategies. The focus should be targeted to this cohort due to their higher rates of hypertension.

Although substantial work has been done to improve conditions, decrease hypertension, and address the health disparities that exist for African Americans in the United States, these disparities persist. Research shows that race and ethnicity are the origins of social disparities in health. Hicken et al. (2014) report that numerous studies have been done to understand what has caused these disparities. But, despite efforts to eliminate them, they continue, even after addressing socioeconomic status, as well as behavioral and biomedical risks factors. The hypertension disparity for African Americans has increased over the past 20 years (Hicken et al., 2014).

Hicken et al. (2014) believed that other factors might be the driving force for racial and ethnic disparities in hypertension. The researchers obtained data from the Chicago Community Adult Health Study by surveying 3105 adults,

18 years of age and over, from 2001 to 2003. This was a cross-sectional survey carried out on black, Hispanic, and white adults that looked at the association between anticipatory stress, otherwise called racism-related vigilance, and the prevalence of hypertension among these three groups.

The study found that blacks commonly reported the highest levels of vigilance, more than white and Hispanic people. The vigilance behaviors reported for blacks was 14 percent higher than the levels reported by the other groups. For instance, black people were prepared for more weekly insults, whereas the behavioral percentage reported by Hispanics was 5 percent, and the lowest by white people at 2 percent.

Hypertension prevalence was positively related to vigilance in black individuals but not whites. The prevalence was 49 percent among blacks, 33 percent for whites, and 32 percent for Hispanics. Surprisingly, the vigilance was so significant and positively linked to hypertension that for a one-point increase in the vigilance scores, the likelihood would be a 4 percent increase in the probability of hypertension. They further reported that racism-related vigilance is a vital determinant of hypertension in black people and probably Hispanics. This is because the stress response system, such as the autonomic and hypothalamic-pituitary-adrenal systems is activated continuously. Whenever these systems are frequently activated, it causes them to be dysfunctional.

Hicken et al. (2014) reported that despite the low vigilance score noted in Hispanics compared to blacks, there was a similar positive relationship between hypertension prevalence and vigilance in this ethnic group.

The findings of Hicken et al. (2014) indicate that the stress of racism-related vigilance combined with its anticipatory and perseverative qualities is a vital contributor to racial disparities in hypertension prevalence. They also believe that when people anticipate discrimination, this may be a key source of stress and "the vigilance for prejudice may be a contributing factor to racial and ethnic health disparities" (p. 122). It is the researchers' belief, based on their study, that focus should not be only directed to conventional risk factors to eradicate the disparities in hypertension, given that there was no change in their study results when there was an adjustment in hypertension risk factors, such as smoking, physical activity, drinking alcohol, diabetes status, and BMI.

Therefore, the need to further address the reasons for health disparity may be crucial since *Healthy People 2010* reported that over the previous ten years, there had been no change in racial or ethnic disparities for 69 percent of the *Healthy People* outcomes that were monitored. In fact, there was a 15 percent increase for these outcomes (Hicken et al., 2014).

The findings suggest the need for more research and preventive intervention measures, especially in the black communities in the United States. These measures may help to decrease prevalence of hypertension and hopefully eliminate the disparities that plague this unfortunate group. This will no doubt improve the health outcomes of black people, decrease the burden of hypertension-related consequences, and decrease economic costs and even mortality rates. While disparities in racism exist, other factors and influences in different countries contribute to disparities.

In a study comparing hypertension prevalence, awareness, treatment and control in England, the United States and Canada, the mean systolic blood pressure was higher in England than in the United States and Canada. While mean diastolic blood pressure was similar in these countries for subjects up to age 50, it fell more rapidly in the United States after age 50. Only 34 percent of subjects had a BP below 140/90 compared with 50 percent in the United States and 66 percent in Canada. Prehypertension and stages 1 and 2 hypertension prevalence figures were also the highest in England. Hypertension awareness was also higher in both the United States and Canada than in England (Joffres et al., 2013).

Statistics of Hypertension, Mortality, and Morbidity—A Brief Overview

An estimated one billion people worldwide have hypertension (Ma et al., 2011). Approximately 9.4 million deaths in a given year may be caused by hypertension and its complications (World Health Organization, 2015). Among rural Indian men, the prevalence of hypertension is low—a shocking 3.4 percent—in comparison to Polish women, which is high at 72.2 percent (Erem, Hacihasanoglu, Kocak, Deger, & Topbas, 2008).

According to the Centers for Disease Control and Prevention (CDC, 2015), about one in three adults in the United States, an estimated 70 million people, have high blood pressure. This figure has increased since 2007, when approximately 65 million Americans were affected (Coly et al., 2008). In 2008 alone, high blood pressure was the primary or contributing cause in more than 347,000 American deaths. Ma et al. (2011) also reported that hypertension is the main cause of morbidity and mortality, and is a public health problem in most countries.

Not only is high blood pressure a contributing factor in increased mortality, it is also costly. The CDC stated that "high blood pressure was projected to cost the United States $93.5 billion in health care services, medications, and missed days of work in 2010" (CDC, 2012, p. 1). In 2007, the cost was estimated at $64.4 billion (Coly et al., 2008). Further, the CDC (2012) pointed to high blood pressure as a major risk factor for heart failure, stroke, and kidney disease, and reported that the leading causes of death in the United States are heart disease and stroke.

Likewise, Aekplakorn et al. (2012) also reported that hypertension is a major risk factor for stroke, heart diseases, and renal diseases. Moreover, worldwide death and disability rates attributed to hypertension are enormously high. For instance, 17 million lives are lost worldwide yearly due to cardiovascular disease with 9.4 million of these deaths caused by hypertension (World Health Organization, 2013) The disability-adjusted life year (DALY) represents the sum of the loss of years from the average lifespan and the years of disability attributed to specific disorders. DALY statistics can be used as a measure of population health. DALY represents health gap and measures the state of a population's health compared to individuals who live to their expected lifespan.

Using DALY researchers at Berkeley found that from 1990 to 2010 the United States made substantial progress in improving health. However, morbidity and chronic disability now account for nearly half of the US health burden, and improvements in population health in the United States have not kept pace with advances in population health in other wealthy nations. A number of risk factors have been identified with the highest being dietary risks followed by tobacco usage, hypertension, high body mass index, and lack of physical activity.

As part of their Blood Pressure Project Study, the researchers investigated risk factors from January 2010 through December 2012 in subjects with uncontrolled hypertension. The primary risk factors were identified as African American ethnicity, living alone, and poor medication adherence (Shadden Laboratory, 2014).

Globally, the DALY or lost years attributed to hypertension is 92 million yearly (Aekplakorn et al., 2012). Multicountry data taken between 1980 and 2008 showed a decrease in mean blood pressure in Western countries, but in Southeast Asia and Oceania the trend had increased (Aekplakorn et al., 2012). In terms of disease ranking, hypertension has been the cause of six hundred thousand DALY losses, which is 6.6 percent each year in Thai people. The authors further postulated that stroke is among the most prevalent of DALY losses in the Thai group, due in part to hypertension. Systolic hypertension is mostly seen in people with hypertension over 50 years of age, "and is more predictive of an impending cardiovascular event than diastolic hypertension in this age group" (Munger, 2010, p. 872). Munger reports that in China, 200 million individuals have hypertension, and it is the most prevalent health problem in adults. For example, the incidence of hypertension has increased to 27.04 percent in adults and 48.8 percent in people older than 65.

Manifestation of Hypertension (Pathophysiology)

There are changes that take place in the body when people have hypertension. The physiological changes of essential hypertension outlined in Madhur et al. (2014) describe the processes in essential hypertension. First, the pathogenesis of essential hypertension is said to be multifactorial and highly complicated. For sufficient tissue perfusion (the oxygenation and delivery of nutrients to capillary beds by blood), multiple factors play a role in modulating blood pressure. Included are humoral mediators, vascular reactivity, circulating blood volume, vascular caliber, blood viscosity, cardiac output, blood vessel elasticity, and neural stimulation.

Madhur et al. (2014) suggest a possible pathogenesis of essential hypertension. They believe multiple factors, such as genetic predisposition, excess dietary salt intake, and adrenergic tone, may interact to cause hypertension. They further point out that although genetics is believed to give rise to essential hypertension, the exact mechanism has still to be determined.

Several hypertension mechanisms have been described. First, in high output hypertension, the results are from a "decreased peripheral vascular resistance and concomitant cardiac stimulation by adrenergic hyperactivity and an altered calcium homeostasis" (Madhur et al., 2014, p. 2). The second mechanism shows a normal reduced cardiac output and elevated systemic vascular resistance. These are caused from an increase in vasoreactivity. The third mechanism is considered to be overlapping. In this mechanism, the kidney reabsorbs increased salt and water (salt sensitivity). This caused an increase in circulatory blood volume (Madhur et al., 2014).

Norris et al. (2008) state that the pathophysiological basics for the predisposition of hypertension and hypertension-related complications in African Americans are evolving, and there is a complex interplay between genetics and environmental factors. According to Norris et al. (2008), salt intake, heavy metal exposure, and stress levels are interplay environmental factors. The authors consider the increase in the prevalence of salt sensitivity in Caribbean and American blacks of African origin a major pathophysiological reason for the vast severity and frequency of hypertension, compared with whites and native black Africans.

Sodium Sensitivity

Norris et al. (2008) suggest that the slave trade from Africa to the Caribbean and the Americas sped up the gene selection for retaining sodium. Sodium retention prevented depleted volume and cardiovascular collapse related to diarrheal diseases and limited supply of drinking water, and thereby "favored the survival of avid sodium retainers" (Norris et al., 2008, p. 539). Individuals who were able to retain more salt were better able to survive the long voyage from Africa to the Americas and Caribbean.

Even though other studies showed no relationship between hypertension and the 24-hour excretion of sodium and potassium in 291 city-dwelling black South Africans, Norris et al. (2008) emphasized that the theory is consistent. As the study showed, African slave descendants' salt sensitivity rate was higher compared to native black Africans.

Genetics

Kaplan (1998) also pointed to genetics and the salt hypothesis in the development of hypertension, and the slavery hypothesis in blacks. Kaplan (1998), in his view on the role of genetics and hypertension, reported that genetic factors may have contributed to hypertension. He further stressed that these factors have been recognized for years. He stated that hypertension clustered in families, with the stronger contributor being the father. Kaplan (1998) emphasized that the final phenotype is blood pressure, which resulted from "the complex impact of environmental influences on the expression of a number of genes" (Kaplan, 1998, p. 42).

The gene is expressed at a subcellular level, and it is changed by other genetic and environmentally conditioned influences. This occurs at four different levels: cellular, tissue, organ, and the final whole-body level (Kaplan, 1998).

In keeping with hypertension and genetics in blacks, Kaplan (1998) reported that polymorphisms in genes for the alpha-2 receptor, angiotensinogen and 11-beta-hydroxysteroid dehydrogenase type 2 are believed to be genetically associated.

A variation is also believed to play a role in the ethnic differences in hypertension prevalence rates. This is especially so for salt-sensitive hypertension and chronic kidney disease. Norris et al. (2008) postulated that the T594M variant to the amiloride-sensitive epithelial sodium channel B-subunit was linked with an increase in sodium retention that occurred almost mainly in black people. Even though the link was strong between the polymorphism and hypertension in a population of black South Londoners, this was not so for a cohort of South African people of African descent, French Afro-Caribbeans, Jamaican blacks, or African Americans. The authors concluded that such observations may suggest the interactions of different polymorphisms and hypertension, and gene environment may be responsible for salt-sensitive high blood pressure. This is among American and European blacks of African descent in comparison to native black Africans.

Other genetic factors may contribute to salt-sensitive hypertension in ethnic individuals. These genetic factors are an increase in function mutations of epithelial sodium channels as seen in Liddle syndrome "or subtle mineralocorticoid excess states, such as glucocorticoid-remediable aldosteronism" (Norris et al., 2008). Genetic variants or polymorphisms such as hyper expression of transforming growth factor B and altered expression of vasoregulatory peptides may have caused hypertension and or the rapid growth of CKD in ethnic individuals (Norris et al., 2008).

Natural History of Essential Hypertension

This type of hypertension develops from occasional or sporadic to established hypertension. But following a long invariable asymptomatic period, continuous hypertension develops into complicated hypertension (Riaz et al., 2011). In this process, target organ complications are seen.

How Complicated Hypertension Affects Target Organs

Complicated hypertension affects target organs such as the aorta and small arteries, heart, kidneys, retina, and central nervous system. This progression starts in different age groups and hypertensive stages (Riaz et al., 2011).

Table 2.
Causes of Secondary Hypertension

Causes

- Renal: (2.5%-6%)
- Parenchymal diseases and renal vascular diseases
  Polycystic kidney disease
  Chronic kidney disease
  Urinary tract obstruction
  Renin-producing tumor
  Liddle syndrome
- Vascular
  Coarctation of aorta
  Vasculitis
  Collagen vascular disease

Causes

- Endocrine: most common
  (1%–2%)
  Exogenous **or** endogenous hormonal imbalances
  Exogenous (from outside the body) causes
- Drugs and toxins
  Alcohol
  Cocaine
  Cyclosporine, tacrolimus
  Steroids including hormones
  Nonsteroidal anti-inflammatory drugs (NSAIDs)
  Erythropoietin
  Adrenergic medications
  Decongestants containing ephedrine
  Herbal remedies containing licorice or ephedrine
  Endogenous (naturally occurring) Causes
  Adrenal hyperplasia
  Kidney diseases
  Hyperthyroidism and hypothyroidism
  Hypercalcemia
  Hyperparathyroidism
  Acromegaly
  Obstructive sleep apnea
  Pregnancy-induced hypertension

Adapted from Madhur et al., 2014.

Table 3. Causes of Primary Hypertension

Environmental or Genetic: Accounts for 90–95 Percent of Adult Cases

Other causes:

- 11-beta-hydroxylase and alpha-hydroxylase and alpha-hydroxylase deficiencies
- Liddle syndrome
- Glucocorticoid-remediable hyperaldosteronism
- Syndrome of mineralcorticoid excess
- Pseudohypoaldosteronism type II

Adapted from Madhur et al., 2014.

According to Madhur et al. (2014), endocrine causes from using oral contraceptives are the most common form of secondary hypertension. Estrogen compounds account for 1 to 2 percent of secondary hypertension. Oral contraceptive risk factors that are believed to be associated with hypertension "include mild renal disease, familial history of essential hypertension, age older than 35 years, and obesity" (Madhur et al., 2014, p. 3). These include exogenous or endogenous hormone imbalances. They postulate that the administration of steroids is included in exogenous causes, while endogenous hormonal causes include primary hyperaldosteronism, Cushing syndrome, pheochromocytoma, and congenital adrenal hyperplasia. Exogenous administration of other steroids such as thyroid hormone and the therapeutic use of nonsteroidal anti-inflammatory drugs (NSAIDs) also increases blood pressure.

Variation in Rates of High Blood Pressure by Age, Gender, and Race

The CDC (2015) reported that women are as likely as men to develop HBP during their lifetimes. For individuals under the age of 45, high blood pressure affects men more than women, and for 65 years and older, more women than men are affected. Table 4 shows this variation by age and gender.

This suggests that women and men of all ages should take measures to prevent high blood pressure, and those at risk should be proactive in detecting hypertension. Based on these statistics, men younger than 45 years old should be more vigilant, as should women 65 years and older.

As illustrated in Table 5, hypertension is higher in African American men and women, compared to other groups.

Table 4.
Rates of High Blood Pressure by Age and Gender

Age Group	*Men (%)*	*Women (%)*
20–34	11.1	6.8
35–44	25.1	9.0
45–54	37.1	35.2
55–64	54.0	53.3
65–75	64.0	69.3
75 & older	66.7	78.5
All	34.1	32.7

Adapted from CDC, 2012.

Table 5.
Rates of High Blood Pressure by Race and Gender

Race	*Men (%)*	*Women (%)*
African Americans	43.0	45.7
Mexican Americans	27.8	28.9
Whites	33.9	31.3
All	34.1	32.7

Adapted from CDC, 2012.

Brief Overview: Role of the Heart in Blood Pressure

The heart plays a key role in maintaining blood pressure, whether an individual has high blood pressure or not. However, individuals with high blood pressure have systolic pressure levels and/or diastolic pressure levels that are higher than those who do not have high blood pressure. It is necessary to know the difference between systolic and diastolic pressures to better understand how the heart works in terms of blood pressure. For this purpose, systolic and diastolic pressures are explained below.

Systole is defined as "the contraction phase of a cardiac cycle" (Spence & Mason, 1987, p. 911) while systolic pressure is "the pressure that is generated by the left ventricle during systole" (Spence & Mason, 1987, p. 911). "Diastolic pressure (diastole = dilation) is blood pressure during the period between heart contractions, when the heart relaxes, dilates, and fills with blood" (Spence & Mason, 1987, p. 526).

Measurements of the systolic and diastolic pressures at different intervals assist the health-care practitioner in determining the individual's diagnosis. "Blood pressure of 140/90 or higher is considered hypertension" (Sentry Health Monitors, 2012, p. 1). Therefore, if the arterial blood pressure is above 140/90 mm Hg, the heart has to pump harder. This is because the systolic and diastolic pressures have an effect on the mean arterial pressure (Spence & Mason, 1987). "Arterial blood pressure (P) is the force excreted by the blood against the arterial wall and it is directly related to the cardiac output (Co) and peripheral vascular resistance" (Kavanagh, 1987, p. 1074).

This suggests hypertensive people need to adhere to treatment regimens to maintain normal blood pressure readings, thus decreasing their chances of developing cardiovascular complications. It is also important for people with normal blood pressure to maintain a healthy lifestyle and have their blood pressure monitored by a healthcare practitioner periodically. This is especially significant for people susceptible to developing high blood pressure. Early detection and treatment of hypertension and other risk factors have contributed to the gradual decline in morality due to heart disease and stroke in high-income countries over the last three decades. Unfortunately, however, nearly 80 percent of deaths due to to cardiovascular disease occur in low- and middle-income countries (World Health Organization 2013). Although it is not within the scope of this book to outline all the functions of the heart, clearly the heart plays a significant role in blood pressure.

Position of the Heart

The adult heart is described as a "cone-shaped" organ. It is about the size of a fist and it is situated between the lungs in the mediastinum space (Spence & Mason, 1987). Figure 2 shows this position.

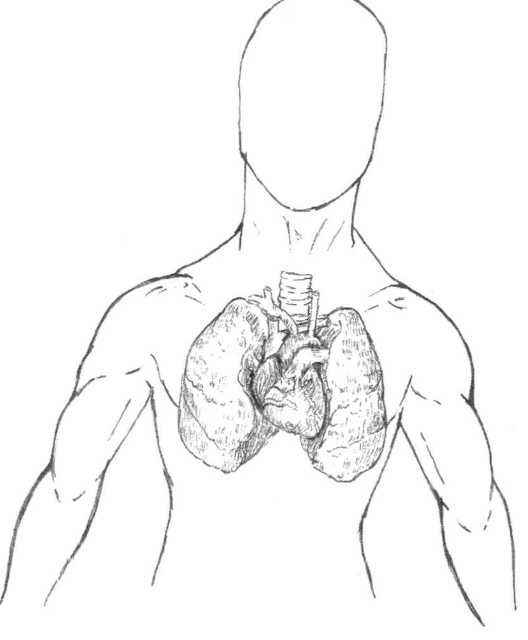

Figure 2. The frontal position of the heart as it is situated in the human body (courtesy Dominique Diedrick).

3

Cardiovascular Disease

Taking adequate control of your blood pressure is one of the key ways to maintain a healthy heart.

The control and management of hypertension are the most important measures for decreasing complications attributed to high blood pressure. This is especially true for African Americans. As Flack et al. (2010) found from their International Society on Hypertension in Blacks (ISHIB) report, effective blood pressure control in this group is a grave necessity.

The ISHIB 2010 consensus highlighted the significance of addressing the broader issues that are important in "the prevention, diagnosis, risk stratification, and clinical management of hypertension and cardiovascular-renal risk reduction in black patients with hypertension" (Flack et al., 2010, p. 781).

In the consensus, Flack et al. (2010) reviewed the applicable hypertension and cardiovascular disease (CVD) treatment and prevention guidelines. The following factors were also considered in this approach:

- Hypertension clinical trials reporting clinical end points, also those undertaken solely in blacks and undertaken with sizeable numbers of blacks;
- Clinical trials that involved hypertension treatment in persons with comorbidities, e.g., diabetes mellitus and chronic kidney disease; and
- The results of hypertension clinical trials in blacks that focused mainly on lowering blood pressure.

In terms of clinical trials that involved treatment for hypertension in people with comorbidities, the study's conclusion emphasized that even though the race of trial participants wasn't reported, these trials of hypertension treatment were carried out in disease states that disproportionately affect black individuals and magnified the risks of pressure-related complications (Flack et al., 2010).

Flack reported that the possibility of formulating a set of comprehensive hypertension treatment guidelines specific to blacks based primarily on randomized trial data only or predominately on this group was not feasible. As a result, Flack et al. (2010) extrapolated results from randomized trials that were carried out in predominately non-black individuals when similar data were unavailable in black individuals.

Therefore, in an effort to appropriately manage hypertension in the black population, the updated consensus statement was based on the interpretation of the blood pressure response and clinical end-point data. They believed the observations from these data fit with the totality of evidence that were available for consideration.

The updated 2010 consensus statement outlined a comprehensive overview of hypertension in the black culture. It detailed the strategies that would be successful in efforts to improve blood pressure and protect target organs in black patients. It is important to note that the updated consensus placed great emphasis on a comprehensive assessment and appropriate risk stratification for individual blacks with hypertension. Flack et al. (2010) stated that practitioners should diagnose individuals, stratify risk, and treat blacks individually, instead of making blanket extrapolations in regard to preferred antihypertensive medications to all blacks.

The JNC 8 guidelines for the treatment of hypertension include recommendations for antihypertensive medications based on age, racial demographics and co-existing conditions. The evidence review in establishing these guidelines included studies with the following subgroups: diabetes, coronary artery disease, peripheral artery disease, heart failure, previous stroke, chronic kidney disease (CKD), proteinuria, age, sex, racial and ethnic groups and smokers (James et al., 2014).

The need for persistent blood pressure monitoring, changing blood pressure medications as needed, and reinforcing overall lifestyle changes are necessary regardless of the pharmacological agents utilized or the specific subgroup, thus ensuring attainment and persistent maintenance of blood pressure below target levels (Flack et al., 2010). Flack et al. (2010) believe that these measures, combined with a greater awareness of hypertension by patients are important for effective control of blood pressure and improved outcomes of all individuals with hypertension.

Studies repeatedly show that African Americans are affected more from hypertension. They develop the disease earlier, and their rates of hypertensive complications such as chronic kidney disease (CKD), stroke, and heart disease are greater compared to their white counterparts (Norris et al., 2008). This is consistent with the findings of Fernandez et al. (2011), who also found that

African Americans are disproportionately affected by hypertension compared to whites when considering its prevalence, treatment, and control rates. The cardiovascular benefits of controlling the disease are also well-documented (Fernandez, et al., 2011).

These findings suggest the necessity for effective blood pressure control and early intervention therapy in the African American population. These strategies will no doubt delay or prevent cardiovascular complications and even mortality attributable to hypertension.

Home Blood Pressure Monitoring

Research shows that high blood pressure is believed to be a modifiable risk factor for heart disease, cerebrovascular disease, and renal diseases. Even though there are effective treatment options for the disease, the rates of hypertension control could be improved. The CDC reports that about 52 percent of people with high blood pressure have their condition under control (CDC 2015). This statistic includes people with hypertension who may not yet have been diagnosed and treated. In the study of hypertension in England, Canada and the United States, among individuals treated for hypertension (i.e., taking medication to lower blood pressure), the proportion being controlled is lowest in England (53 percent) compared with 71 percent in the USA and 82 percent in Canada (Joffres et al., 2013).

These statistics are staggering and a cause for concern. Improving the quality of hypertension care should be the main priority to sustain individuals' health and prevent hypertension related consequences.

Although it is necessary for hypertensive people to undergo regular follow-up visits with their primary practitioners for blood pressure control and to decrease their risks of hypertension complications, a recent commentary showed a progressive reduction in the availability of primary care in adult groups in the United States.

This reduction has threatened the possibility of better control of risk factors and lessens the opportunities for cardiovascular disease prevention (Krakoff, 2011). This is why technology such as home blood pressure monitoring (HBPM), combined with telemedicine, may play a key role in improving control of hypertension (Krakoff, 2011). According to this author, HBPM offers one pathway for expanded diagnosis and treatment of hypertension; this may decrease the demand for clinic visits. It is also noted that in prospective surveys, home blood pressures were better correlated with long-term cardiovascular outcomes compared with clinic pressures.

There are electronic, mercury and aneroid devices that are used to measure blood pressure. The World Health Organization (WHO) recommends the use of affordable and reliable electronic devices that have the option to select manual readings. Semi-automatic devices enable manual readings to be taken when batteries run. Because mercury is toxic, EHO recommends that mercury devices be phased out in favor of electronic devices. Aneroid devices such as sphygmomanometers should only be used if they are calibrated every six months and used by individuals who have been trained in their use (World Health Organization 2013). While most devices measure systolic and diastolic blood pressure as well as heart rate, some devices such as the Bioclip Cuff also measure vascular condition, which is linked to arterial flexibility, an important risk factor for assessing the likelihood of heart attack or stroke (Millasseu et al, 2002).

Krakoff (2011) stated that more than 50 percent of patients in hypertensive households in the United States have a blood pressure device, and that extensive literature for HBPM has pointed out evidence of the importance of this device. The author believes that the fast growing acceptance of Internet and wireless communication facilitates the development of widespread use. These systems also have the potential for linkages to electronic health records that are now required for patient care in the developed nations (Krakoff, 2011).

The benefits of HBPM are also documented to be an effective tool compared to clinic visits. According to Krakoff (2011), the benefits of HBPM are

- easier documentation in patient medical records;
- more effective review to improve care with a single-source database;
- small but significant decrements in treatment of systolic and diastolic blood pressure compared with usual management of hypertension; and
- enhanced education and feedback from nurse clinicians or pharmacists providing support through phone calls, emails or Web-based communications.

Negative Outcomes of Clinic Visits Versus Home Blood Pressure Monitoring

According to Krakoff (2011), clinic visits are inconvenient and costly for patients, especially working patients or those with daily responsibilities. "Working patients find it difficult to take time off of work for visits" (p. 791), it takes time to travel to clinics or offices, and the cost of travel (e.g., increased gas prices) is a barrier to care.

Self-Management for Hypertension Using Home Blood Pressure Monitoring

Self-management of anti-hypertensive medications combined with HBPM has also been examined as a method to improve control of hypertension. Krakoff (2011) stated that in the first report of the self-management approach, patients were taught an algorithm for changing medication and using HPBM diaries for reporting. In this approach, 20 participants were managed by self-titration with HBPM and 11 with usual care. The result showed that during eight weeks, there was an approximate 1mm Hg small reduction in systolic pressure in the intervention group and a small, approximately 2 mm Hg, increase occurred in the control group.

Krakoff (2011) points to "the Telemonitoring and Self-Management in the Control of Hypertension" (TASMINH2) trial. This trial "compared HBPM telemetry combined with self-management (263 participants) and usual care (264 participants) from general practices in the United Kingdom"(Krakoff 2011, p. 793). Objective office pressures at baseline and 12 months were used as study parameters.

The findings showed a greater reduction in both systolic (-5.4 mm HgP < .004) and diastolic pressure (-2.7 mm HgP < .001) in participants of the intervention group than those in the usual care group.

Krakoff (2011) points to the concept of evidence-based support for self-management of hypertension, because this approach has been broadly accepted for diabetes management. It is Krakoff's belief that "HBPM with transmission of results to providers, together with opportunities for self-management, offers a vista of a major potential for increased control of hypertension for patients healthy enough so that frequent office visit/clinic visits are not needed" (p. 793).

Krakoff (2011) also emphasized the hurdles to this approach. However, Krakoff believes the acceptance by providers and patients of HBPM as a method of monitoring blood pressure is promising. The author further stated that in the TASMINH2 trial, 71 percent of patients who used HBPM together with self-titration preferred this management approach compared with only 41 percent who preferred usual care.

Krakoff (2011) concluded that an optimistic approach to the wide use of technology can defeat the increasing deficits in numbers of primary care providers. This is partially the case in the U.S. to guard the health of individuals at risk for cardiovascular diseases "in decades to come" p. 794.

The use of HBPM is worth pursuing given the prevalence of hypertension, especially in the U.S. population. Further research needs to be conducted in the African American communities with the use of HBPM devices. Given the benefits of this approach, the implementation of this device in homes may very well help to decrease risks of cardiovascular diseases attributed to hypertension.

In a similar clinical trial study by Magid et al. (2013), the authors pointed out the benefits of HBPM with the use of the pharmacist-led American Heart Association's Heart360 online monitoring tool, in comparison to usual care (UC) for patients with blood pressure that was not controlled. Their purpose was to find out whether patients randomly placed in the HBPM intervention group would have greater blood pressure control than those patients randomly placed in the UC group.

The study was conducted at Kaiser Permanente Colorado (KPCO) in ten primary clinics throughout Colorado. Each of these clinics had more than one clinical pharmacy specialist on staff. These specialists provided assistance with the management of drug therapy to primary care providers and worked under a preapproved collaborative drug therapy management program, which empowered them to start or change antihypertensive medications, adjust dosages and order lab tests.

At the KPCO, clinicians utilized a commercial EpicCare electronic health record (EHR) which is a routine method of providing care at the clinics. One feature of the KPCO electronic health record, called "My Chart," enables communication between patients and providers through a password protected website.

For this study, adult patients ages 18 to 79 were eligible if they were diagnosed with hypertension and their blood pressure was above the recommended level, which meant two recent clinic blood pressure readings were above goal systolic blood pressure of 140 mm Hg or diastolic blood pressure of 90 mm Hg. Individuals with diabetes mellitus or chronic kidney disease had systolic blood pressure greater than 130 mm Hg or diastolic blood pressure greater than 80 mm Hg. Also, to be included in the study, the patients were required to have less than three prescribed antihypertensive medications, have a primary care provider working at one of the ten participating clinics, and be registered on the Kaiser Permanente website, demonstrating Internet access.

Baseline study clinic visits were carried out between October 2008 and November 2009 on patients who had shown interest by not submitting the opt-out postcard that was mailed to them. At the clinic visit, blood pressure was measured and patients with mean blood pressure that was above their goal were eligible to participate in the study.

Of the 348 patients, 175 were assigned to the HBPM group and 173 to the UC group. Those in the HBPM group were instructed in how to use a blood pressure cuff (Omron HEM-790IT) that fit properly. Individuals were also required to measure their blood pressure three times a week, and were to upload their blood pressure readings onto their Heart360 account on a weekly basis. In addition, HBPM patients were provided with written educational material, which listed information about diet, physical activity, and how to manage high blood pressure.

More information on the use of the Heart360 web application can be found at https://www.heart360.org/Default.aspx

Patients assigned to the UC group were also given educational information on diet, physical activity, and how to manage high blood pressure. After being informed that they had high blood pressure the UC patients were advised to follow up with their primary care physicians. Additionally, the UC group patients' physicians were informed about their elevated blood pressure.

Clinical pharmacy specialists weekly reviewed HBPM group blood pressure readings, as well as its members' adherence to taking the prescribed medication. It was also the responsibility of the clinical pharmacist specialists to contact patients after reviewing weekly summary reports of their HBPM reading averages, and to note those with blood pressure averages above their usual. Medication adjustment was done if required and patients were notified either by telephone or secure email. Physicians were updated about changes in medication.

Of the enrolled study participants, 326 completed the follow-up visit at six months. Twenty-two patients (thirteen from the HBPM group and nine from the UC group) did not. Of the patients that did follow up, 162 were in the HBPM group and 164 were in the UC group.

The mean age of the study population was 60 years; forty percent of participants were female, 83 percent were white, and almost half (49 percent) had diabetes mellitus (DM) and chronic kidney disease (CKD).

At the six-month follow-up, patients' blood pressure was measured. They were asked to rate their hypertension care in terms of their satisfaction and how much they were occupied in their hypertension care for the six months.

Those in the HBPM group were asked whether it was easy to take their blood pressure in their homes, how easy it was to upload their measurements to the website and to provide ratings of how the clinical pharmacy specialists interacted with them.

The study revealed that at six months, patients in the HBPM group had achieved greater blood pressure improvement than the UC group. Improvement was seen in 54.1 percent of patients in the HBPM group and 35.4 percent of patients in the UC group. The mean blood pressure after 6 months was lower in the HBPM group than in the UC group. For instance, the SBP was 128.1 mm Hg for the HBPM group versus 137.4mm Hg for the UC group. The DBP was 79.1mm Hg in HBPM patients versus 83.1 mm Hg in UC patients.

In comparison to the UC group, the HBPM group had experienced a larger drop of 12.4 mm Hg in SBP and 5.7 mm Hg in DBP. In the subset of patients with co-existing conditions of CKD and DM, blood pressure lowering interventions were greater. Additionally, in this subset and in the HBPM group, there was a larger drop in both SBP (15.4 mm Hg) and DBP (7.3 mm Hg). Also, within this subgroup of patients with DM and CKD, the proportion of individuals that had accomplished their target BP goal was higher for the HBPM group than the UC group. The percentage of patients achieving their BP goal was 51.7 percent for HBPM versus 21.9 percent for the UC group. However, patients in both the UC and HBPM groups demonstrated SBP and DBP average blood pressure readings that decreased throughout the study period.

It was also shown that patients in the HBPM group had received more e-mail and telephone contacts and a greater medication regimen increase than those in the UC group.

Not only were blood pressure lowering effects noted but a good proportion of the patients stated they "were very or completely satisfied with their hypertension care" (Magid et al., p. 160); the reported satisfaction was 58 percent in the HBPM group and 42 percent in the UC group. The HBPM group also reported greater awareness in terms of paying increasing attention to their blood pressure, with HBPM participants reporting 60 percent compared to the UC group's 40 percent. In addition, 68 percent of those in the HBPM group stated that the blood pressure cuff and the "Heart360 monitoring system were very or extremely easy to use" (Magid et al., p. 161). In rating the clinical pharmacy specialist interaction, 52 percent of the study patients rated their interaction as very or extremely helpful.

The researchers believed their study showed that improvement in blood pressure control can be obtained with HBPM intervention using clinical pharmacy specialists who are experts in the management of medication therapy, such as adjusting doses, adding or stopping antihypertensive medications, and ordering lab tests for adverse reactions. These specialists are also able to summarize blood pressure readings, contact patients with hypertension, and provide valuable feedback in an effort to help patients learn to control their blood pressure.

Magid et al. (2013) pointed out that successful use of the Heart360 Web application is an easy and effective method for patients to send their blood pressure measurements to their clinical pharmacy specialist, instead of having to make extra office visits.

The findings of the Colorado study suggest that HBPM may be an effective tool for individuals with poorly controlled hypertension. Effective application of this intervention can help to decrease health problems strongly linked to uncontrolled high blood pressure. However, this method requires relatively intact cognitive abilities and good eyesight; individuals with these abilities will be better able to see blood pressure numbers and learn the steps to upload their blood pressure readings to the Heart360 application.

The desire for people to control their blood pressure using HBPM intervention also requires patients to be compliant with their medication dosages, especially if the medications require adjustments. They must be motivated and willing to monitor and report their blood pressure measurements as needed. Nevertheless, any application of successful HBPM intervention is worth pursuing if an individual's blood pressure will be better controlled as a result.

Ambulatory Blood Pressure Monitoring

In 2003, the recommendations for blood pressure measurement were published by the working group on blood pressure monitoring of the European Society of Hypertension (ESH). Further guidelines for home blood pressure measurement were published in 2008. O'Brien, Parati and Stergiou (2013) stated that the first meeting of ESH to develop these recommendations, which took place in 1978 in Ghent, looked at the possibility of Ambulatory Blood Pressure Monitoring. Ever since, many conferences regarding the consensus on blood pressure monitoring have been carried out by the ESH working group.

Many individuals may question the significance of ABPM, but Bunker (2014) states that ABPM will rule out individuals with white-coat hypertension. But what is ABPM?

Definition of Ambulatory Blood Pressure Monitoring

According to Bunker (2014), ABPM is the measurement of blood pressure with an automatic monitor while the patient performs activities of daily living. This measurement is carried out for almost 24 hours.

O'Brien, Parati and Stergiou (2013) have outlined the reason for using this device in clinical practice: "to identify untreated patients who have high blood pressure readings in the office but normal readings during usual daily activities outside of this setting, that is, white-coat hypertension, and to identity varying 24-hour blood pressure profiles" (p. 989). The authors reported that the indication is the consensus and is on par with international recommended guidelines.

O'Brien et al. (2013) reported that after consensus regarding the clinical indicators for ABPM was reached, the recommended international guidelines were reviewed. These guidelines were published between 2000 and 2013. "All these guidelines were in agreement that ABPM is indicated for the exclusion or confirmation of suspected white-coat hypertension"(O'Brien et al; 2013, p. 989).

The ESH 2013 ABPM position paper points to the need for the evaluation of ABPM accuracy in specific groups, such as children and patients with arrhythmias. This is because the devices for ABPM have been validated for adults, but for children and patients with arrhythmias validation is not frequently done. As a result, the ESH ABPM position paper has urged manufacturers to broaden validation for this specific group.

Cost-Effectiveness of Ambulatory Blood Pressure Monitoring

According to O'Brien et al. (2013), ABPM is cost-effective. Benefits include ABPM's identification of people with normal blood pressure during doctor office visits but high blood pressure levels in daily life (masked hypertension). Other cost-effective aspects are that ABPM may improve drug prescribing, because it also will identify people with white-coat hypertension and may allow for financial savings in medication prescribing by showing the effectiveness of antihypertensive drugs throughout the course of 24 hours. Even though it was recently reported that ABPM was more expensive than some other measurement techniques, it has been found to be cost-effective in specialist services and primary care. For example, O'Brien et al (2013) claim a possibility for savings of 3 to 14 percent for the cost of hypertension care with the use of this measurement technique.

Furthermore, if ABPM is included in the diagnostic process, there may be a 10 to 23 percent decrease in treatment days, which would yield a yearly cost of less than 10 percent of the treatment costs. In addition, ABPM is specifically "cost-effective for the diagnosis and management of newly diagnosed hypertension" (O'Brien et al; 2013, p. 992).

Importantly, the most recent cost analysis conducted by the National Institute for Health and Care Excellence (NICE) revealed that when ABPM is used, it is the most cost-effective method to confirm hypertension diagnosis in individuals who are suspected of having high blood pressure. This is based on the conventional high blood pressure screening measurement (blood pressure greater than 140/90 mm Hg).

The authors emphasized the need to evaluate the cost-effectiveness of ABPM at an international level, because its use will vary from country to country. This is because the price of ABPM and the management of hypertension is not the same across countries; the method of delivering healthcare is also a factor. It is estimated that the introduction of ABPM in Japan for hypertension management decreased medical costs by 9.48 trillion yen over a ten year period (O'Brien et al. 2013).

But the question is, who should carry out ABPM? According to O'Brien et al. (2013), a great number of individuals with hypertension access primary care for the management of their hypertension. As a result, doctors in this setting may develop ABPM services independently or make referrals to an ABPM service. O'Brien et al. (2013) believe that a pharmacy setting may be appropriate to start the referral of people for ABPM in partnership with primary care physicians or specialists because it is documented that blood pressure control has been improved when pharmacists are "engaged in the management of hypertension" (O'Brien, 2013, p. 993).

It is important to note that the Centers for Medicare and Medicaid Services (CMS) approved the use of ABPM in the United States in 2001, allowing reimbursement for the use of ABPM in identifying people with white-coat hypertension. Additionally, NICE in the United Kingdom made the recommendation in 2011 that every person suspected of having hypertension should be offered ABPM as a cost-effective technique (O'Brien et al., 2013).

A recent study focused on whether blood pressure load, independently of blood pressure level, was associated with target organ damage. Liu et al.'s (2013) cross-sectional study was conducted on 869 participants. Of these, 430 were men with a mean age of 51, and 439 were women. The mean age of the women was not reported. Participants had not taken antihypertensive medications for at least two weeks and were either normotensive (33 percent) or were untreated mildly hypertensive patients (67 percent). Participants completed 24 hours of ambulatory blood pressure monitoring and comprehensive cardiovascular measurements.

For this study, the definition of blood pressure load is the percentage of blood pressure values greater than 135mm Hg systolic or diastolic 85 mm Hg diastolic on readings taken during the day, or 120/70 mm Hg during the night (Liu et al., 2013, p. 1813).

The findings demonstrated that BP load was associated with target organ damage including arterial stiffness, left ventricular hypertrophy and microalbuminuria. On the other hand, BP load was not independent of the 24-hour blood pressure level. Lui et al. (2013) pointed out that their findings supported previous studies, such as the Kirschner and Hamilton (2014) study, which showed a correlation between blood pressure load and target organ damage.

The authors concluded that based on the clinical implication of their findings, focus should be on control of blood pressure level for managing hypertension. Lui et al. (2013) emphasized the need for further studies on hypertensive high-risk individuals in a broader setting. Future studies will determine whether there is a connection "between BP load and hypertension organ damage" (p. 1817).

Reducing Risk Factors of Coronary Heart Disease in Special Populations to Meet Healthy People 2020 Objective

Coronary heart disease (CHD), which is caused by coronary artery disease (CAD), is a common term for the buildup of plaque in the heart's arteries, a condition that could lead to a heart attack. Hypertension is one of the risk factors for CHD. Other risk factors include high levels of low density lipoprotein (LDL) cholesterol, low levels of high density lipoprotein (HDL) cholesterol, family history, diabetes, smoking, being post-menopausal in women and age over 45 years in men. Obesity may also be a risk factor. Children of parents with heart disease are more likely to develop CHD. African Americans have more severe high blood pressure than Caucasians and consequently have a higher risk of CHD. Heart disease risk is also higher among Mexican Americans, American Indians, native Hawaiians and some Asian Americans. This is partly due to higher rates of obesity and diabetes (American Heart Association, 2016).

The CDC (2011) reported that the "age-adjusted mortality rates for CHD have declined steadily in the United States since the 1960s" (p. 2084). Multiple factors may have played a role in the decline of CHD deaths in the United States. The control of risk factors has been the major contributing factor in this decline. Increased control of risk factors and improved treatment have resulted in a decline in CHD deaths (CDC, 2011). It is believed that improved treatment would actually increase the prevalence of CHD, because when treatment lowers death rates more people are living with CHD.

An analysis of data from the Behavioral Risk Factor Surveillance System (BRFSS) surveys completed between 2006 and 2010 was conducted in the United States to estimate the prevalence and recent trends in CHD. This estimate was a state-specific approach conducted by the CDC in 2011 to gather data about CHD prevalence and recent trends specific to age, sex, race and ethnicity, and education.

Hispanics, whites, blacks, Asians, Native Hawaiian and Other Pacific Islanders and American Indian and Alaskan Natives were surveyed. This survey was carried out in 50 states, with participants 18 years and older. The number of study respondents ranged from 347,790 in 2006 to 444,927 in 2010 and included subjects from all states.

The result of the analysis revealed that overall, self-reported CHD prevalence in the United States had declined from 2006 to 2010 from 6.7 percent to 6.0 percent, although there were substantial differences in prevalence by age, sex, race and ethnicity, education, and the state in which individuals had resided (CDC, 2011).

The decline in CHD prevalence was observed among whites and Hispanics from 2006 to 2010. The decline was from 6.4 percent to 5.8 percent for whites and from 6.9 percent to 6.1 percent for Hispanics. Substantial differences in prevalence based on the age of subjects were observed. For instance, in 2010, CHD prevalence was greatest among individuals older than 65; next, aged 45 to 64 years, followed by individuals aged 18 to 44 years. In comparison, the greater prevalence of the disease was observed in men than women (7.8 percent versus 4.5 percent). The prevalence of CHD was also greater among individuals who had less than a high school education (9.2 percent) compared to those who had graduated from high school (6.7 percent), those with some college education(6.2 percent), and individuals who had acquired postgraduate education (4.6 percent).

In 2010, the prevalence of CHD among racial/ethnic populations was greatest in American Indians/Alaskan Natives, second, in blacks, third Hispanics, then whites, followed by Asians or Native/Hawaiians Other Pacific Islanders. For example, the prevalence of CHD was 11.6 percent in American Indians/ Alaskan Natives; in blacks 6.5 percent; in Hispanics 6.1 percent; in whites 5.8 percent, and in Asians or Native Hawaiians/Other Pacific Islanders 3.9 percent.

In terms of race and gender, the prevalence was greatest in male American Indians/Alaskan Natives (14.3 percent) and whites (7.7 percent). Among females, the greater prevalence was seen in American Indians/Alaska Natives at 8.4 percent, followed by blacks at 5.9 percent (CDC, 2011). The CDC (2011) reported, "By state, from 2006–2010, the greatest statistically significant linear declines in age-adjusted CHD prevalence were 23.1 percent in West Virginia (from 10.4 percent to 8.0 percent) and 22.1 percent in Missouri (from 7.7 percent to 6.0 percent)" (CDC 2011, p. 2085).

A person's education level was also shown to be a key factor. For example, as stated earlier, CHD prevalence was greater in people with less than a high school education. This result may suggest that the less education an individual has, the greater the chance of developing CHD. However, further studies need to be conducted to evaluate the effects of CHD prevalence and education levels in different age groups and genders.

According to the CDC (2011), despite five states demonstrating an increase in the prevalence of the disease between 2006 and 2010, there were no statistically significant linear increases in any of these five states. The CDC (2011) emphasized that data from this evaluation would assist health planners in creating targeted prevention programs. This would include states with populations that had a greater prevalence of CHD, for example, states with a higher male American Indian/Alaska Native population and female black population.

Importantly, "development of effective prevention programs targeting populations with greater CHD prevalence should reduce risk factors and CHD incidence, which will continue the decline in both CHD prevalence and CHD deaths" (CDC, 2011, p. 2086). The CDC also states that the information gathered by surveys will allow state and national health agencies to monitor the prevalence of CHD. This would assist in the progression toward the achievement of the Healthy People 2020 objectives—to reduce the 2020 mortality rates from CHD in the United States by 20 percent from the 2007 baseline.

Hypertension and Its Relation to Left Ventricular Hypertrophy

Left ventricular hypertrophy (LVH) refers to an enlargement and thickening (hypertrophy) of the walls of the heart's main pumping chamber (left ventricle). Left ventricular hypertrophy can develop in response to various factors such as high blood pressure or other heart conditions that cause the left ventricle to work harder. This subclinical cardiovascular disease is shown to be one of the strongest independent indicators of cardiovascular morbidity and mortality in the general population (Wang et al., 2011).

Even though it is documented that both hypertension and LVH are more prevalent in blacks in comparison to whites, there is inconsistency in data regarding high blood pressure levels and the close association with increased LV mass in studies involving these two groups. Also, there is limited literature on the effect of blood pressure levels and its influence on LVH geometry and remodeling in both black and white young adults.

In an effort to understand the effects of blood pressure and LV geometric patterns in asymptomatic young black and white adults, Wang et al. (2011) conducted the Bogalusa Heart Study, a biracial, community-based investigation of the early nature of cardiovascular disease. A combination of echocardiography and cardiovascular risk factor measurement was utilized for this study of 1,123 subjects, of which 780 were white and 343 were black. All participants were 24 to 47 years of age and lived in Louisiana; 42.2 percent of the subjects were men. Subjects' blood pressure was measured in a sitting position using the right arm. Systolic and diastolic blood pressure were recorded at the first and fifth Korotkoff phases with a mercury sphygmomanometer, and the results were determined by the average of the six blood pressure readings.

Importantly, recorded blood pressure values were adjusted for 147 subjects who took medications for hypertension. The adjustments were a 10 mm Hg addition to the systolic blood pressure and a 5 mm Hg addition to the diastolic blood pressure. These adjustments were determined by the average expected treatment effects. The authors had identified the following four LV geometry types for this study:

- Normal
- Concentric remodeling
- Eccentric
- Concentric hypertrophy

Wang et al. (2011) also defined four different patterns of LV geometry. These were "normal LV geometry, normal relative wall thickness with no LV hypertrophy; concentric remodeling, increased relative wall thickness but no LV hypertrophy" (p. 718). In addition, cholesterol and triglyceride serum levels were assayed with the use of enzymatic procedures. Glucose levels were also measured as part of a multiple chemistry profile (SMA2) with the use of enzymatic procedures.

The study revealed a greater prevalence of eccentric hypertrophy in blacks compared to their white counterparts, and in concentric hypertrophy the prevalence was also greater in blacks than in whites. For instance, the prevalence of eccentric hypertrophy was 15.7 percent in blacks while in whites, it was 9.1 percent. In blacks, the prevalence of concentric hypertrophy was 9.3 percent and in whites it was 4.1 percent. Nevertheless, only systolic blood pressure was associated with concentric hypertrophy in white subjects. Neither black or white subjects blood pressure levels were associated with concentric remodeling.

Regarding body mass index (BMI), black and white subjects both had BMIs that showed consistent associations with eccentric hypertrophy and concentric hypertrophy, but no association with concentric remodeling. Being female was associated with a lower risk of concentric remodeling, but it was more likely for female subjects to have concentric hypertrophy—especially black females.

The prevalence of hypertension was greater in black individuals (33.2

percent vs. 15.1 percent, $p <.001$). Black hypertensive subjects' SBP was higher (143.8 mm Hg) compared to white hypertensive subjects (135.7 mm Hg). Similarly, the average DBP in whites was 94.3 mm Hg while in blacks it was 95.5 mm Hg.

"The mean BMI levels, lipid variables, glucose levels, and blood pressure did not differ significantly between the normal geometry and concentric remodeling groups" (Wang et al; 2011, p. 719).

In comparison, the roles of obesity and the relation of blood pressure to LVH were more pronounced in whites than in blacks. This study showed the differences among blacks and whites in the pathogenesis of LV hypertrophy and its potential role in developing cardiovascular disease. The researchers also concluded that if the disparities of the pathophysiologic basics of LVH by race and ethnicity were better understood, such knowledge would encourage both clinicians and public health professionals to develop and implement preventive programs, carry out interventions that are culturally sensitive, and provide services that are aimed at risk burdens in different populations.

According to Peterson et al. (2013), hypertensive African Americans are at higher risk of adverse results from cardiovascular and renal disease. For blacks cardiovascular-related illnesses and deaths are also higher in the United States. Given that African American people are at higher risk, it would be beneficial to target this population.

Prevalence of Cardiovascular Disease (CVD)

A vast number of studies show the prevalence of cardiovascular disease in the population, and these studies also indicate specific groups that are most likely to be affected by this condition. One of the contributing risk factors for cardiovascular disease is hypertension. The CDC (2015) reports that approximately 70 million Americans, or close to an estimated 1 in 3 adults, have high blood pressure. DeVore (2010) also stated that 29 percent of adults in the United States have hypertension, and the CDC (2015) reports that the percentage of controlled blood pressure among this population is 52 percent. In the United States, "CVD is the leading cause of death" (Powell-Wiley et al., 2012, p. 99). This is consistent with Cardarelli et al. (2010), who also stated that CVD is a chief cause of death in adults and that as many as 70 million people are affected in the United States.

African Americans are believed to be disproportionally afflicted due to elevated risk factors in their population. For instance, Powell-Wiley et al. (2012) reported that cardiovascular risk factors such as hypertension, hyperlipidemia, and obesity affect African Americans at greater rates, which leads to a higher burden of CVD.

The death rates from CVD are a cause for concern, especially in developing countries. Dramatic decreases in death rates from this disease occurred some time ago in Finland and the United States, and studies have highlighted some of the factors that led to that decline. For instance, Chiha, Njeim and Chedrawy (2012) reported that the estimated 47 percent decrease in death rates from CVD in the United States between 1980 and 2000 was due to advancements in medical therapies and treatment gains in coronary syndromes and heart failure, while almost 44 percent of the reduction was due to secondary factors, namely declines in such cardiovascular risks as hypercholesterolemia, hypertension, smoking, and physical inactivity.

In 1972 in North Karelia, in Finland, residents had an extremely high mortality rate from heart disease. Within 5 years a reduction in coronary disease was observed as a result of dietary changes, improved hypertension control, and smoking reduction. As a result these changes were implemented in national programs. Thirty-five years later, observed reductions in serum cholesterol, blood pressure and smoking and programs to reduce salt consumption have resulted in an 85 percent reduction in mortality resulting from cardiovascular disease (World Health Organization, 2013). However, this scenario is not the same in developing countries.

The rapid evolvement of the CVD epidemic on a global level is presently the cause for "twice as many deaths in developing countries when compared to developed countries" (Chiha et al., 2012, p. 1). CVD is presently the cause of 30 percent of all deaths worldwide, and most of the burden is presently taking place in developing countries (Chiha et al., 2012). Death is a major result of the impact of CVD worldwide, but disability from this condition is also a significant factor. For example, disability-adjusted life years (DALYs) were 58 million (Gaziano et al., 2010). The World Health Organization (2013) reports that CVD accounts for approximately 17 million deaths annually, nearly one third of the total. Of these, complications of hypertension account for 9.4 million deaths worldwide every year.

Gaziano et al. (2010) reported that three-fourths of global deaths and 82 percent of total DALYs that are correlated with CHD were in low and middle income countries. In 2007, deaths from cardiovascular disease accounted for 33.7 percent of all deaths worldwide compared to other chronic diseases, for example, "cancer, 29.5 percent, other chronic diseases 26.5 percent, injury 7 percent and communicable diseases 4.6 percent" (Gaziano et al.; 2010, p. 73).

CVD death rates in high-income countries are estimated to be 38 percent.

In contrast, "the overall rate of CVD deaths is 28 percent in low- and middle-income countries, which ranges from a high of 58 percent in Eastern Europe to a low of 10 percent in sub-Saharan Africa" (Gaziano et al., 2010).

The population that is most affected is young people residing in developing countries, representing a staggering 80 percent of the estimated 16.7 million cardiovascular deaths worldwide (Gaziano et al., 2010). The premature deaths in this young population of productive members of the workforce pose a significant threat. This impact is felt on both the families and economies of less-developed countries, where there are limited resources. Although CVD is believed to be the largest cause of death in all developing regions except sub-Saharan Africa, the leading cause of death in sub-Saharan Africa, infectious disease, affects people over 45 years old (Gaziano et al., 2010).

The causes of heart failure are due to several conditions: coronary artery disease, hypertension, and dilated cardiomyopathy. These conditions occur in an extensive proportion of people in the Western world (Hunt et al., 2005). According to Peralta and others (2014), people over the age of 75 are the fastest growing group in the United States, and two-thirds of this population has high blood pressure. High blood pressure is a risk factor for cardiovascular diseases and mortality in this specific demographic (Peralta et al., 2014). Arterial hypertension has been linked to a high risk of cardiovascular illnesses and death. Furthermore, many studies frequently demonstrate a high frequency of cardiovascular complications in people with resistant hypertension, when compared to those without resistant hypertension (Weitzman, Chodick, Shalev, Grossman, & Grossman, 2014). The condition of resistant hypertension is discussed in Chapter eight.

Definition of Heart Failure

Heart failure is a complex clinical syndrome arising from any cardiac disorder, whether structural or functional, which weakens the ability of the ventricle to fill with blood or force out blood (Hunt et al., 2005). The human heart is illustrated in Figure 3.

Hunt et al. (2005) reported that heart

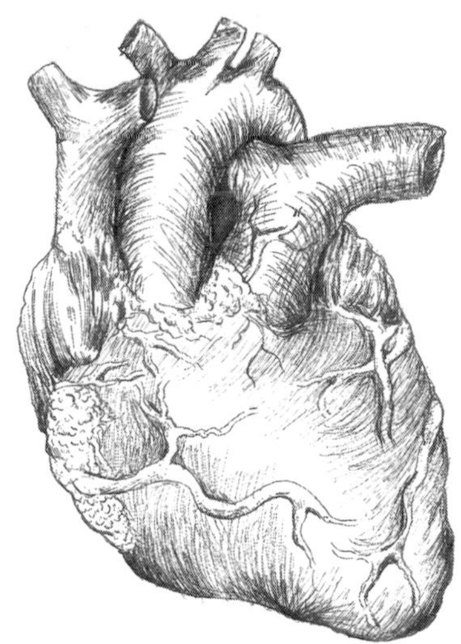

Figure 3. A human heart in the anterior position. The right and left coronary arteries supply oxygenated blood to the heart muscle (courtesy Dominique Diedrick).

failure is a great public health concern in the United States and he explains that increased heart failure in the elderly population contributes a great deal to the overall incidence of heart failure, because this condition is mainly seen in elderly people. Additionally, treating people with heart failure is costly. For example, Hunt et al. (2005) stated that "Medicare diagnosis-related groups (e.g., hospital discharge diagnosis), and more Medicare dollars are spent for the diagnosis and treatment of heart failure than for any other diagnosis" (p. 1827). Take, for instance, the spending cost in the United States. In 2005, it was estimated that the direct and indirect costs of heart failure amounted to $27.9 billion, and medications for treating heart failure cost the government almost $2.9 billion a year (Hunt, 2005)

This figure is huge. Given the estimated number of people with heart failure in the United States, the treatment cost could further increase if measures are not taken to decrease risk factors. According to Hunt et al. (2005), nearly five million people in the United States have heart failure, and more than 550,000 people are newly diagnosed with this condition every year. The death rate is also high. For example, in 2001 almost 53,000 patients died with heart failure reported as the main reason. The authors strongly believe that health providers should identify people at risk for developing this disease by paying special attention to the four stages of development of heart failure syndrome.

Stages of Heart Failure

Heart failure progression consists of stages A, B, C, and D. In Stages A and B individuals have preliminary conditions that would put them at risk for developing heart failure. For example, in Stage A, people may have conditions such as "coronary artery disease, hypertension or diabetes mellitus, who do not yet demonstrate impaired left ventricular function, left ventricular hypertrophy (LVH) or geometric chamber distortion" (Hunt, 2005, p. 1827). In Stage B, people exhibit no symptoms, but show LVH and/or have impaired left ventricular function. Stage C applies to people who presently have heart failure symptoms or have had symptoms of heart failure that have been linked with an underlying structural heart disease. Lastly, in Stage D, are individuals who have true refractory heart failure and may be considered eligible for specialized advanced treatment, such as procedures to help with the removal of fluid or cardiac transplantation.

Hunt et al. (2005) stated that the main risk factors for the development of heart failure in individuals are elevated blood pressures, especially systolic blood pressure. They further stated that the long-term treatment of both blood pressure levels showed a reduction in heart failure risk.

Heart Failure in Ethnic Minority Populations in Canada

Heart failure is also a major concern in Canada and other countries. According to Moe and Tu (2010), Statistics Canada 2006 census data revealed that visible minority groups have exceeded five million, bringing them to 16.2 percent of the total population. In the province of Ontario, Chinese, South Asians, blacks, and people of aboriginal descent accounted for over 1.5 million people. Moe and Tu (2010) emphasized the importance of understanding cultural differences and social environments in managing heart failure. These authors assert that hypertension is the reason for heart failure in Asian, African, and African American groups, and that the incidence of heart failure prior to the age of 50 in African Americans has been linked to hypertension, obesity, chronic kidney disease, and systolic dysfunction. African Americans are more likely to experience heart failure than their white counterparts. Nevertheless, coronary artery disease and uncontrolled blood pressure in both white and African American people are the highest risk factors (Mo and Tu, 2010).

Mo and Tu (2010) reported that the greater burden of coronary artery disease in South Asians may have given rise to their high prevalence of heart failure. Mo and Tu (2010) pointed to a study comparing South Asians and whites who were hospitalized with heart failure. The study revealed South Asian individuals had experienced a similar rate of prior coronary artery disease, but their mortality rates were lower. Nonetheless, both hypertension and diabetes occurred more often in South Asian people than whites. Furthermore, Mo and Tu pointed to a retrospective sequential chart review, which involved South Asians and non–South Asian whites who were hospitalized at two Toronto community hospitals with heart failure. It showed that when it came to diabetes, although the South Asians were younger with lower BMI, diabetes was more common in this population than in non–South Asian white patients.

Mo and Tu (2010) further reported the incidence of heart failure in Chinese patients, pointing to a study that showed hypertension was one of the major risk factors for the 730 Hong Kong Chinese patients admitted to hospitals with heart failure. Similarly, high blood pressure was often the reason for heart failure in all age groups of women. These authors also referred to another subsequent study reported by the same group, carried out on 200 consecutive individuals with heart failure, that utilized Doppler echocardiography. It showed that more than 45 percent of left ventricular ejection fraction was normal, whereas vascular heart disease was shown in 12.5 percent of individuals.

According to Mo and Tu (2010), "The Study of Health Assessment and Risk Evaluation in Aboriginal Peoples (SHARE) reported a higher frequency of CVD among aboriginals in Canada and a greater burden of atherosclerosis when compared with Canadians of European ancestry" (p. 128). The authors believed that along with the higher rates of diabetes that come with aboriginals being transitioned from a traditional lifestyle to a more urban one, it is likely that CVD incidence will increase in this group, and consequently, heart failure.

This finding suggests the need to recognize and understand the social changes, socioeconomic statuses or experience, and individuals' perceptions of their illnesses. This can be achieved by listening to their views and understanding their perceptions. It is also pivotal that the level of communication be understandable. At the same time, care should be provided in a manner that is culturally sensitive, ensuring a positive experience and outcome. Healthcare providers, policy-makers, agencies, government, and communities all play a role in implementing policies, guidelines, and providing education and services to manage the conditions of individuals with heart failure. The focus should not only be in Canada but also in other countries or populations—particularly in the United States, where there are wide variations in ethnic backgrounds. These strategies may help to decrease prevalence of heart failure in vulnerable populations, thus helping ethnic minorities to live healthier and longer lives. It would be worthwhile to conduct similar research on a larger cohort of ethnic minorities both in Canada and the United States to compare the differences.

Role of Diabetes and Coronary Artery Disease

Mounting data has shown a rising prevalence of diabetes and its impact on health and the population as a whole. Somewhat similarly, the prevalence of hypertension is also reported to be high in persons with diabetes (Yamout, Lazich & Bakris, 2014). The health outcome of individuals with diabetes is concerning not only in North America but worldwide. This is because whenever someone has type 2 diabetes he or she is also at a higher risk for developing cardiovascular disease. This can lead to increased death rates, illness, and costs (Crowley et al., 2013). It is estimated that 180 million people in the world have diabetes mellitus, and it is expected that this amount will double by 2030 (Gaziano et al., 2010).

Of these individuals with diabetes mellitus, 90 percent are afflicted with type 2 diabetes. Gaziano et al. (2010) further reported that approximately 80 percent of individuals with type 2 diabetes reside in low- and middle-income countries. They stated that the eventual increases in this condition are projected to be higher in Asia, Latin America and the Caribbean, and sub-Saharan Africa, and that the rate of growth will exceed 104 percent to 162% percent whereas in the United States, the growth rate will be approximately 72 percent and in Europe 32 percent. Furthermore, the authors report that most individuals with this disease are affected between age 45 and 64 in the developing countries. In contrast, people 65 and over will make up the majority in the developed countries.

Hypertension and Heart Disease in Diabetes

The American Diabetes Association (ADA) 2011 standard of medical care in diabetes indicates that a majority of patients with diabetes mellitus have hypertension. In patients with type 1 autoimmune diabetes, kidney disease is often the cause of the hypertension, whereas in patients with type 2 diabetes hypertension is one of a group of related cardiometabolic factors. The standards note that a reduction in blood pressure may result in improved kidney (renal) function. Early detection of microalbumin in urine, which they recommend, is one of the best ways to identify even minor signs of kidney disease. With early detection and aggressive therapeutic interventions for hypertension, the diabetic complication of end-stage renal disease may be prevented (Madhur and Maron, 2014).

Type 2 diabetes has also been shown to be a risk factor for coronary artery disease (Daniels et al., 2013), and Chiha et al. (2012) state that diabetes mellitus is a cardiovascular risk factor in developed countries, reporting that a Framingham study revealed the incidence rate for cardiovascular disease in men with diabetes to be twice that than for nondiabetic men. But in diabetic women, it was three times more elevated when compared to nondiabetic women.

Additionally, the Copenhagen City heart study reported that "the relative risk of incident myocardial infarction was [a twofold to threefold] increase in diabetics compared to nondiabetics. This was independent of the presence of other known cardiovascular risk factors such as hypertension" (Chiha et al., 2012, p. 2). Nevertheless, there is differential impact of diabetes in relation to coronary artery disease deaths in women and men (Chiha et al., 2012). The author further pointed out that the "relative risk of coronary artery disease" death in women is 2.5, and 1.85 in men.

This study shows that regardless of other risk factors and gender, individuals diagnosed with diabetes mellitus in developed countries need to be proactive and take interest in their health to delay or prevent the development of heart disease. Communities and government also play important roles in implementing strategies to better serve their communities, thus ensuring the improved health of everyone.

Developing countries also experience great challenges in terms of diabetes and its role in cardiovascular disease. Even though research about the relationship between diabetes mellitus and cardiovascular disease originated mainly from studies conducted in European-origin populations, rising data gathered from other ethnic groups and emerging countries also identify diabetes as one of the major contributors of the worldwide epidemic of cardiovascular disease (Chiha et al., 2012).

Chiha et al. (2012) initiated the INTERHEART study, a case control study that included 52 patients from different countries in a representation of all inhabited continents. The purpose was to assess whether there was an association between acute myocardial infarction and a variety of risk factors, including diabetes mellitus, and if there were variations based on geographic region, ethnic origin, or age. The findings showed that of the nine risk factors, diabetes was one factor that was significantly related to acute myocardial infarction. This was shown in all age groups and both genders in all regions of the world. In addition, the population considered at risk for only diabetes showed 9.9 percent in the total study population.

Some Coronary Artery Changes in People with Diabetes and Whether Vitamin D Deficiency Plays a Role

There is an increase in the prevalence of coronary plaques in the hearts of people with diabetes, and these plaques are at high risk for rupturing. According to Chiha et al. (2012), a coronary angiography and angioscopy study showed that in 55 consecutive patients admitted to the hospital with unstable angina, 94 percent of the patients with diabetes had ulcerated plaque, compared to only 60 percent in nondiabetics. In addition to these plaque observations, thrombi were noted in the same percentage (94 percent) of individuals with diabetes, compared to 55 percent thrombi presence in nondiabetics (Chiha et al., 2012).

In a similar postmortem study of coronary atherectomy specimens carried out on 47 percent diabetic and 48 percent nondiabetic patients, it was shown that the arteries of patients with diabetes had higher lipid content and increased macrophage infiltration, as well as thrombosis (Chiha et al., 2012). The authors believe that even though multiple mechanisms may play a role, hyperglycemia (high blood sugar) is often the trigger.

Freedman et al. (2010) pointed to ethnic differences in the development of calcified atherosclerotic plaque (CP) in European Americans and African Americans. They reported that the physiological changes in calcium and phosphorus metabolism in individuals may be due to ethnic differences. The authors further stated that the inclusion of the markedly low amounts of CP in African Americans is a related phenomenon, although there is a greater presence of conventional CVD risk factors. These observations have led Freedman et al. (2010) to theorize that biological ethnic differences may be factors in the processing of bone and vascular health. When a person consumes calcium and phosphorus, it is absorbed in the gastrointestinal tract. Vitamin D plays a significant part in this absorption, and allows proper maintenance of bone health (Freedman et al., 2010). According to these authors, vitamin D deficiency is more prevalent in African Americans, compared to European Americans. Lower levels of 25-hydroxyvitamin D in people has been linked to diabetes, subclinical atherosclerosis, hypertension and inflammation.

Freedman et al. (2010), in their American Diabetes Heart Study, evaluated 340 unrelated African American individuals with type 2 diabetes. The group consisted of 140 males and 200 females who were diagnosed with diabetes after age 30. The study sought to determine whether there was any association between "circulating vitamin D and quantitative measures of CP [calcified atherosclerotic plague] in three vascular beds, four organ-specific adipose tissue depots, and vertebral BMD [bone mineral density] in the thoracic and lumbar spine" (Freedman et al., 2010, p. 1080).

Blood calcium levels are known to be regulated by parathyroid hormone and vitamin D. In the study, the circulating form of vitamin D, highly sensitive C-reactive protein (hsCRP), which is a marker of inflammation, and intact parathyroid hormone (PTH) were measured. The authors also determined the region of adipose tissue volumes, CP, and thoracic and lumbar vertebral bone density with the use of a computed tomography (CT). Furthermore, they assessed the relationships between organ-specific adipose tissue and vascular CP in relation to vitamin D, CRP, and intact PTH.

Three different imaging tests were used for the study. These were vascular imaging, adipose tissue imaging, and bone imaging. The measurement of calcified atherosclerotic plaque was done in the coronary, carotid, and infrarenal abdominal aorta arteries. For adipose imaging, pericardial adipose tissue (PAT) and visceral adipose tissue (VAT) were measured from volumetric CT acquisitions. Regarding bone imaging, "Quantitative CT for volumetric trabecular bone mineral density (BMD); milligrams per cubic centimeter of the thoracic and lumbar vertebrae were measured" (Freedman et al., 2010, p. 1078). This measurement was performed using images acquired for CP in the coronary and abdominal aorta as well as an external calibration phantom as in prior reports.

The study showed a positive association between serum 25-hydroxyvitamin D concentrations and both carotid artery CP, and infrarenal aorta CP in the subjects with diabetes. However, the association was negative for coronary CP in African American subjects. No noticeable association between highly sensitive C-reactive protein and CP, visceral adipose tissue, pericardial adipose tissue, subcutaneous adipose tissue, or bone density was noted in this study of African Americans with diabetes.

According to Freedman et al. (2010), calcified atherosclerotic plaque confirms the presence of subclinical atherosclerosis, and coronary artery CP can be used as a predictive factor of cardiovascular events in the future for European Americans, Asian Americans and African Americans. However, the researchers stated that their findings in relation to 25-hydroxyvitamin D and subclinical atherosclerosis are unique when it comes to African Americans.

They believe their findings have contradicted what was previously detected in subjects of European backgrounds. For instance, studies of Amish, European American (Health Professionals Follow-Up Study), and Italian individuals showed that "25-hydroxyvitamin D concentrations are inversely associated with subclinical atherosclerosis as measured by CP or carotid intima-media thickness" (p. 1080).

Freedman et al. (2010) questioned whether 25-hydroxyvitamin D supplement would be beneficial for African Americans with a deficiency in this vitamin for cardiovascular health. Furthermore, the direct correlation between this important vitamin and the amounts of CP in African Americans may be different, when compared to a European-derived group of individuals. This is because a lower level of vitamin D is believed to cause exorbitant risks for atherosclerotic cardiovascular disease and osteoporosis in European groups.

The authors believe that the effects of supplementation of vitamin D on atherosclerosis in African Americans with vitamin D insufficiency or deficiency remains uncertain. The general recommendation is that people with vitamin D levels lower than 74.9 nmol/L (30 ng/ml) require supplementation (Freedman et al., 2010). This is because supplementation with vitamin D_3 is believed to play a role in protecting people from osteopenia and osteoporosis, serving as a treatment for these two conditions, as well as benefiting cardiovascular health (Freedman et al., 2010).

They concluded that there is a need for future large-scale longitudinal studies of African Americans to quantify the levels of vitamin D and its association with adiposity and CT-derived CP. Also, the need to determine the normal range of blood concentration of 25-hydoxyvitamin D, as this level may vary between different ethnicities and needs to be addressed in the African American population.

Lee Goldman, MD, explains that the low vitamin D levels found in people with dark skin (higher melanin content) are due to genetic mutations that allowed individuals to conserve the B vitamin, folate, at the expense of vitamin D. As people migrated to colder climates, this change has resulted in an epidemic of vitamin D insufficiency and deficiency in this population (Goldman, 2015: 20–5).

Biochemical Changes in Diabetes

Some biochemical changes resulting from hyperglycemia are increased reduction of nicotinamide adenine dinucleotide (NAD+) to NADH and increased production of uridine diphosphate (UDP) N-acetylglucosamine. Although NADH is believed to be an oxidative stressor at the cellular level, so far it has not been proven. Nevertheless, UDP N-acetylglucosamine is believed to change enzymatic cellular function (Chiha et al., 2012).

Diabetic Atherosclerosis

Glycosylation of protein (reaction of protein and glucose molecules) in the arterial wall of an individual is thought to cause diabetic atherosclerosis. In the meantime, nonenzyme reactions between glucose and proteins in the arterial wall develop "in the formation of advanced glycation end products" (Chiha et al., 2012, p. 2).

The formation of advanced glycation end products intensifies with hyperglycemia. It is also presumed these end products directly interfere with endothelial cell function and this interaction tends to speed up atherosclerosis.

Diabetic Coronary Plaque

Hyperglycemia also results in increased formation of reactive oxygen species. When reactive oxygen species are formed, they prevent the endothelial production of nitric oxide (NO), and they stop the movement of vascular smooth muscle cells into the intimal plaques. This step is important in order to stabilize coronary plaques. As a result, the risk of coronary plaques rupturing rises (Chiha et al., 2012).

What Happens If a Plaque Ruptures?

If a plaque is ruptured, increased thrombogenesis and platelet dysfunction are notable in the diabetic individual. Thus, clinical consequences of plaque rupture get worse. During this stage, the floating glucose molecules enter platelets freely, causing "an increase in intracellular glucose concentration and progress to the activation of protein kinase C, decreased platelet derived NO, and increased expression of glyclprotein Ib, a platelet aggregation mediator" (Chiha et al., 2012, p. 2). This process may give rise to the intensified thrombosis in diabetic individuals (Chiha et al., 2012).

Heart Disease Risk Factors

People can be at risk for heart disease with or without high blood pressure. However, high blood pressure is widely documented to be a major risk factor (Aekplakorn et al., 2012). Other reported risk factors confirmed in other studies are type 2 diabetes (Crowley et al., 2013; Daniels et al., 2013; Powell-Wiley et al., 2012), hyperlipidemia, obesity (Powell-Wiley et al., 2012), vitamin D deficiency (Harris, 2011), infections, toxins (e.g., alcohol or drugs) and conditions that are inherited (White et al., 2014).

A Health Professionals Follow-Up Study was conducted by Cahill et al. (2013) in 1992. Participants included 26,902 American health professional males, ages 45 to 82, with approximately 97 percent of the participants being of white European descent, with neither cardiovascular disease nor cancer. Test subjects included dentists, veterinarians, pharmacists, optometrists, osteopaths, and podiatrists. This prospective analysis was undertaken to determine whether eating habits and skipping breakfast were connected to an increased risk of coronary heart disease (CHD).

The authors found that during the 16-year follow-up, there were 1,527 reported diagnosed cases of CHD. It was shown that men who skipped breakfast and men who regularly ate late at night had an increased risk of CHD, and these were linked to body mass index (BMI) and other health-related mediated conditions, namely, hypertension, hypercholesterolemia, and diabetes mellitus. In contrast, there was no association with how often participants ate and CHD risk.

According to Cahill et al. (2013), other studies have revealed that eating habits have been associated with many CHD risk factors. These risk factors include being overweight, dyslipidemia (blood lipid disturbances), hypertension, and insulin sensitivity (Cahill et al., 2013, p. 340). CHD has also been linked to diabetes mellitus and mortality.

The authors concluded that eating breakfast was associated with a lowered risk of CHD (p. 342). However, they stated that since their study was the first to be carried out on the relationship of eating habits and CHD, it would require replication. The replication would be beneficial for women and other nonwhite individuals. Additional studies are needed to provide information about the risk of CHD in women and nonwhite individuals.

4

Vitamin D

What Is Vitamin D and How Is It Metabolized?

Vitamin D is a fat-soluble vitamin that can be found in the forms of vitamin D_2 and vitamin D_3. Vitamin D_2 is also called ergocalciferol, and it originates from plants. Humans do not make vitamin D_2. Vitamin D_3 is also called cholecalciferol, and it is obtained from exposure to the rays of the sun and from eating certain foods (Khara, 2010). Vitamin D_3 is the recommended form of supplementation (Moyad, 2009). Two ways in which vitamin D_3 treatment can be administered are through vitamin D_3 supplementation or exposure to UVB radiation (Pilz et al., 2011).

The primary way to produce vitamin D is through skin exposure to the sun's ultraviolet rays (Van Horn et al., 2011). The ultraviolet light reacts with unprotected skin, allowing it to produce vitamin D (Khara, 2010). The concentration of 25-hydroxyvitamin D (25 OH vitamin D), which is the form recommended for blood test measurements, can increase with increased exposure to sunlight. "Sunlight-induced vitamin D synthesis in the skin can be equivalent to a daily vitamin D supplementation of up to 10,000 to 20,000 IU [international units]" (Pilz et al., 2011, p. 580). It is important to note that the skin's ability to make vitamin D lowers with age and some people have mutations to the vitamin D receptor that prevent them from absorbing sufficient vitamin D.

When vitamin D enters the body's circulation, it is changed in the liver to 25 OH Vitamin D (Harris, 2011). 25 OH Vitamin D is converted in the kidney to the most biologically active metabolite, 1,25-dihydroxyvitamin D (Harris, 2011, p. 1175S). While a blood test for 1,25-dihydroxyvitamin D is available, it is not used routinely to measure vitamin D status although this test has value in cases when serum calcium level is elevated or an individual has a disease that might produce excess amounts of vitamin D, such as sarcoidosis or some forms of lymphoma (because immune cells may make 1,25-dihydroxyvitamin D). Rarely, this blood test may also be indicated when abnormalities of the enzyme that converts 25-hydroxyvitamin D to 1,25-dihydroxyvitamin D or renal disease are suspected. Levels of 1,25-dihydroxyvitamin D are also increased in patients on antibiotic therapy as a result of Herxheimer reactions.

Functions of Vitamin D

Vitamin D has many crucial functions in the body and is believed to play a significant role in human growth and development. It also helps in the maintenance of a healthy immune system (Khara, 2010). Studies have pointed to the benefits of vitamin D and its impact on skeletal health, but it also has been documented to protect against chronic health conditions. For instance, various forms of vitamin D are believed to protect against inflammatory and autoimmune conditions, such as "periodontal disease, Sjogren's syndrome, type 1 and type 2 diabetes, multiple sclerosis, and rheumatoid arthritis" (Harris, 2006, p. 1128). Khara (2010) points to similar benefits of vitamin D.

- Maintains normal calcium and phosphorus levels, thus helping maintain and build strong bones, teeth, and nails
- Supports cell functions and other neuromuscular functions
- Supports bone mineralization by hardening them and building and breaking down bone (osteoblasts and osteoclasts)
- Prevents rickets in children and prevents osteoporosis and osteomalacia in adults
- Helps in combating depression, prostate and breast cancer, high blood pressure, cardiovascular diseases, phagocytosis activity, and boosts antitumor activity
- Helps in the treatment of diabetes and obesity, and helps prevent the onset of multiple sclerosis

Because vitamin D plays such vital roles in the body, it would be beneficial for people to absorb this vitamin through sun exposure, food sources, or supplements. Studies have shown that a low mean plasma concentration of 25 OH Vitamin D is more pronounced in black Americans than white Americans (Palmer-Thierry et al., 2008), which is consistent with Harris (2006), who also found lower rates of 25 OH Vitamin D in African Americans, occasionally lower than what is typically found in other American groups.

However, low vitamin D levels are found in all ethnic and age groups for a variety of reasons, including genetic mutations, other compounds that react with the vitamin D receptor (low levels are typically seen in both men and women on androgen or hormone deprivation treatment for prostate cancer or those on this or a similar medication for other medical conditions), and aging. In his update on Vitamin D, Moyad (2009) writes, "To my knowledge, no group in the world consistently carries a higher than normal vitamin D blood level. This is true for African Americans, Asians, Caucasians, Hispanics, babies, pregnant women, adolescents, older adults, and middle-aged individuals."

Individuals with vitamin D deficiency have been found to have a high risk for certain other conditions. For instance, studies show that "vitamin D deficiency may be an important risk factor for cardiovascular disease and type 2 diabetes" (Harris, 2011, p. 117S). Vitamin D deficiency is also linked to other health conditions, such as "cardiac hypertrophy, hypertension, prostate cancer, osteoporosis, and decreased muscle strength" (Palmer-Thierry, 2008, p. 278).

Does Vitamin D Play a Role in the Development of Hypertension?

"Low vitamin D levels, measured as 25 OH Vitamin D, the main circulating form, have been associated with incident hypertension, insulin resistance, peripheral arterial disease, cardiovascular disease, and mortality" (Melamed, Astor, Michos, Hostetter, & Powe, 2009, p. 2631). Most clinical laboratories use the following definitions for Vitamin D insufficiency and deficiency:

- A normal level of vitamin D is defined as a 25 OH Vitamin D concentration greater than 30 ng/mL (75 nmol/L).
- Vitamin D insufficiency is defined as a 25 OH Vitamin D concentration of 20 to 30 ng/mL (50 to 75 nmol/L).
- Vitamin D deficiency is defined as a 25 OH Vitamin D level less than 20 ng/mL (50 nmol/L)

Different conditions are associated with vitamin D deficiency and vitamin D insufficiency. The most serious complications of vitamin D deficiency are related to hypocalcemia, which is a condition of low blood calcium; hypophosphatemia, which is a condition of low blood phosphate; rickets (softening of the bones that commonly occurs during childhood); and osteomalacia, which is a softening of the bones in adults. However, these complications have become less common over time because many foods and drinks have added vitamin D.

Vitamin D insufficiency (also known as subclinical vitamin D deficiency) is frequently seen during routine blood testing and does not usually cause any visible signs or symptoms. However, vitamin D insufficiency often results in reduced bone density (osteopenia or osteoporosis), and in some cases a mild decrease of the blood calcium level, elevated parathyroid hormone (which accelerates bone resorption), an increased risk of falls, and possibly fractures, all of which can seriously affect a person's quality of life (Drezner, 2016).

Judd, Nanes, Ziegler, Wilson and Tangpricha (2008) conducted a cross-sectional study from 1988 to 1994 using data from the Third National Health and Nutrition Examination Survey, which studies the health of the civilian, noninstitutionalized U.S. population older than 2 months of age. The analysis was limited to adults in the United States. The National Center for Health Statistics, Centers for Disease Control and Prevention obtained the data. Field clinic visits at mobile examination centers and household interviews were used to collect findings. The aim of the Judd et al. (2008) study was to determine whether there was an association between blood pressure and circulating 25 OH Vitamin D in black and white adults. This study examined 7,699 individuals who were never told that they had hypertension. Subjects were 47 percent male and 53 percent female; of these, 39 percent were black and 61 percent white. Most of the individuals (79 percent of blacks, 63 percent of whites) were less than 50 years of age. The authors utilized a 25 OH D cutoff point of less than 80 nmol/L to define vitamin D insufficiency.

The findings showed a significant inverse association between circulation 25 OH vitamin D concentrations and systolic blood pressure category in both white men and women. White individuals with lower 25 OH Vitamin D concentrations had higher blood pressure categories, ranging from normotensive to mildly hypertensive. When age was considered, the age-associated rise in systolic blood pressure was lower in white individuals whose circulation concentrations of 25 OH Vitamin D were greater than 80 nmol/L compared to their black counterparts with less than 50 nmol/L. However, significantly lower concentrations of 25 OH Vitamin D were noted in both black males and females at all levels of blood pressure classifications, compared to their white counterparts.

However, there was no inverse association between 25 OH Vitamin D and blood pressure classifications in black males and females. An alarming 92 percent of black individuals' concentration of 25 OH Vitamin D was less than 80 nmol/L, indicating vitamin D insufficiency, whereas only 61 percent of the white subjects showed such levels. Judd et al. (2008) emphasized that black individuals with sufficient amounts of 25 OH Vitamin D were not part of this study's analysis of the U.S. black population, because only 8 percent of blacks' 25 OH Vitamin D concentrations were greater than 80 nmol/L. This led the researchers to analyze only white individuals for 25 OH Vitamin D concentrations greater than 80 nmol/L, which is considered sufficient vitamin D, based on the definition.

Judd et al. (2008) stated that their findings give reason for further studies to see if vitamin D supplements can decrease systolic blood pressure in individuals at risk for developing hypertension. In 2009 one study has shown that calcium and vitamin D_3 supplements can cause a significant decrease in systolic, but not diastolic, blood pressure in elderly females with vitamin D deficiency (Pfeiffer et. al, 2009). However, a meta-analysis of data from multiple studies showed no significant effect on blood pressure. While this is currently an active research topic, individuals should consult with their health practitioners before taking any form of vitamin D supplements (Khara, 2010).

Some Food Sources of Vitamin D

Vitamin D can be found in a variety of foods and in the form of supplements. Some vitamin D food sources are eggs, vitamin D–fortified milk, and fortified cereals (Van Horn et al., 2011). Other food sources are green leafy vegetables, cheeses, sardines, mackerel, salmon, herring, and orange juice (Khara, 2010).

The Connection Between Vitamin D Insufficiency and Blood Pressure: A Comparison

Studies show a strong association between vitamin D levels in the body and differences in blood pressures in blacks and whites. Not only has vitamin D disparity been recognized, but the acknowledgment that suboptimal vitamin D levels are associated with conditions more common in blacks has also been established (Fiscella, Winters, Tancredi, & Franks, 2011). For example, Fiscella et al. (2011) stated that conditions such as peripheral vascular disease, diabetic neuropathy, kidney disease (which progresses to renal failure), and cardiovascular deaths have been associated with suboptimal vitamin D levels in the body.

These authors report that black individuals in the United States have higher age-adjusted blood pressure than their white counterparts. However, the reasons for the difference between the two groups are undetermined.

Fiscella et al. (2011) pointed to a previous study that revealed factors such as diet, social support, stress, and obesity as contributors to the condition. Yet, these factors have not completely explained why black subjects' blood pressure tends to be higher.

Fiscella et al. (2011) set out to answer that question, conducting a cross-sectional study that examined the potential contribution of vitamin D to racial disparity in blood pressure levels. The samples included data collected from

2001 to 2006 on adult non–Hispanic blacks and non–Hispanic whites, aged 20 years and older, by the National Health and Nutritional Examination Survey. Note that systolic blood pressure measurement was only measured for this study because the authors believed systolic blood pressure was more strongly linked with cardiovascular mortality than diastolic pressure (Fiscella et al., 2011).

The findings revealed that vitamin D indeed provides one piece of the complex puzzle concerning race and blood pressure. The findings also contribute broader evidence that links low levels of vitamin D to cardiovascular disparities in black individuals. It was noted that when subjects who took blood pressure medication were removed from the study, levels of 25 OH Vitamin D explained 40 percent of the disparity. Additionally, the study pointed to a vital part of the residual difference in blood pressure among black and white subjects—higher blood pressure level was linked to vitamin C status. Despite utilization of subjects with and without hypertension, the control of multiple confounders, and the use of multiple objective measures, Fiscella et al. (2011) found that lower serum 25 OH Vitamin D levels are a contributing factor to disparities in systolic blood pressure.

The findings from this study suggest a grave need for statewide interventions at a broader level and the need for further studies. This approach may help to decrease the disparities between black and white low vitamin D levels, which put some people at risk for cardiovascular illnesses and even death. If the disparity is minimized, the chances of people developing cardiovascular diseases or even dying from the consequences of disease burden could decrease, and as such, general population health could also be improved.

According to Fiscella et al. (2011), "hypertension is the most important proximal determinant of disparities in cardiovascular disease" (p. 1109). They linked their findings to other studies that have shown low levels of vitamin D in blacks may give rise to cardiovascular disparities. The authors recommended that instituting interventions to reduce disparities could have population-wide impact on rates of heart disease and stroke. They also proposed an urgent need for randomized controlled trials of different age ranges. The authors stated that these trials could test the hypothesis of the importance of vitamin D as a contributor to racial differences in hypertension and cardiovascular health conditions.

Lower Vitamin D Levels and Mortality

Past research has restricted the major health problems stemming from vitamin D deficiency to conditions such as rickets, osteoporosis, and osteomalacia

(Ginde, Scragg, Schwartz, & Camargo, 2009). But new data has emerged, revealing that deficiencies in this important vitamin have been linked to other health problems such as hypertension, diabetes mellitus, and cardiovascular disease (Ginde et al., 2009). Shea et al. (2011) stated that the physiological function of vitamin D goes further than the skeletal system health, which may explain their recommendation for greater vitamin D concentrations. They suggested that 25 OH Vitamin D concentrations greater than 30 ng/ml (75 nmol/L) must be maintained. Further, if this concentration level is maintained, adequate vitamin D levels could be kept consistent. Adequate amounts of vitamin D would help to fulfill both calcemic and noncalcemic demands.

This level is important because a serum 25 OH Vitamin D level of 30 ng/ml or greater has been linked to improved cardiometabolic and functional results (Shea et al., 2011). Studies reveal that more than one-third of the U.S. population shows a deficiency in vitamin D (Judd et al., 2008). The prevalence of vitamin D deficiency is said to be increasing in elderly American adults.

A study conducted by Ginde et al. (2009) evaluated the association between serum 25 OH Vitamin D levels and mortality in a representative U.S. sample of 3,408 Third National Health and Nutrition Examination Survey subjects, all of whom were older adults. Data including age, sex, race, ethnicity, and socioeconomic status was obtained. It is important to note that details related to poverty—"income ratio (the ratio of a family's income to the poverty threshold of a family of the same size)"—was obtained for this study. These individuals were African Americans and Mexican Americans aged 65 and over. They were enrolled from October 1988 through October 1994 and were followed for mortality data until December 31, 2000.

The findings showed an inverse association between the serum 25 OH Vitamin D baseline level and the risk of mortality in noninstitutionalized older adults. There was not only a simple mortality risk but also a strong association of two times greater odds of mortality for those with 25 OH Vitamin D levels less than 25 nmol/L, "independent of demographics factors and other common CVD and mortality risk factors" (Ginde et al., 2009, p. 1597). Pilz et al. (2011) stated that apart from cardiovascular disease, a deficiency in this vitamin is also linked to higher risk of total mortality.

According to the researchers, a stronger association between 25 OH Vitamin D and all-cause mortality in older adults with diabetes mellitus with low baseline 25 OH Vitamin D levels was found, compared to those without diabetes. Among the subjects the median 25 OH Vitamin D level was 66 nmol/L; levels for women, non–Hispanic blacks, and Mexican Americans were lower. Participants with hypertension, a history of stroke, and particular residency (such as the Midwest region) were more likely to have lower levels of 25 OH Vitamin D.

Ginde et al. (2009) stated that the connection between vitamin D and mortality was especially strong in individuals with baseline 25 OH Vitamin D levels less than 25 nmol/L and 25 to 49.9 nmol/L. Additionally, among individuals with diabetes mellitus, low baseline 25 OH Vitamin D levels, older age, and history of stroke and myocardial infarction had a stronger association with cardiovascular disease (CVD) and all-cause mortality (p. 1897). Of interest, lower socioeconomic status, winter season in Midwest regions, and lower physical activity levels were also reported to have an association with lower levels of 25 OH Vitamin D.

The authors stressed that a higher level of 25 OH Vitamin D, for example, 100 nmol/L or more, may be required to improve the survival rates of older adults, given that present recommendations for vitamin D supplement dosages seem to be inadequate for older adults. If supplement dosage is increased to the level suggested, this would increase optimum health levels in this cohort and decrease death rates (Ginde et al., 2009). They also maintained that their findings are consistent with various reports showing a link between vitamin D deficiency, CVD, and CVD mortality risk.

Parathyroid Hormone and Vitamin D Levels

Pilz et al. (2011) stated that increased parathyroid hormone (PTH) levels are linked to higher risk of cardiovascular events and deaths. They pointed to the mechanistic effects of PTH and how it increases blood pressure and exerts many actions on the heart, as well as myocardial hypertrophy and pro-arrhythmic activity. They rightly stated that when PTH is suppressed by the supplementation of vitamin D, it is possible that cardiovascular risk could be decreased. When the concentration of PTH increases, vitamin D decreases; it is clear that the two are closely, yet inversely, connected. As a result, when vitamin D deficiency is being treated, PTH levels will decrease. It may be that greater PTH levels result in higher risk for CVD (Schneider & Michos, 2014). But even though PTH increases may be one mechanism in situations where decreased vitamin D concentration resulted in higher risk of cardiovascular disease through greater vascular remodeling, other mechanisms may have been assumed, such as "activation of the renin-angiotensin-aldosterone system, elevation of blood pressure, adverse glucose/metabolic profile, increased inflammation, and increased atherogenesis" (Schneider & Michos, 2014, p. 1289).

Low Vitamin D Levels and Cardiovascular Disease

A similar study done by Fiscella and Franks (2010) examined whether serum 25 OH Vitamin D deficiency predicted subsequent cardiovascular mortality among U.S. adult subjects, and whether differences in 25 OH Vitamin D levels contributed to black-white differences in age- and gender-adjusted cardiovascular deaths. The researchers obtained data from the nationally representative Third National Health and Nutrition Examination Survey which ran from 1988 to 1994. Subjects were 18 years or older. Fiscella continued to assess cardiovascular death from data collection until December 31, 2000, based on the study's linked mortality file. Subjects were classified as white (non–Hispanic), black (non–Hispanic), Hispanic, and other.

This study showed that 16 percent of the population had 25 OH Vitamin D levels that were in the lowest quartile of the sample studied. It was shown that subsequent higher cardiovascular deaths were associated with lower baseline 25 OH Vitamin D levels. The association seemed "to be partly mediated through cardiovascular-related conditions (hypertension, heart failure, myocardial infarction, stroke, kidney disease, and diabetes)" (Fiscella & Franks, 2010, p. 15). The association was also noticed when multiple cardiovascular risk factors were controlled. It was also established that 25 OH Vitamin D levels were associated with the higher age- and gender-adjusted cardiovascular deaths in black subjects.

In the model that included exogenous variables such as age, gender, month, and region, subjects who were black had a 38 percent higher rate of cardiovascular deaths when compared to white subjects, revealing that low 25 OH Vitamin D levels had been independently predictive of cardiovascular deaths in blacks. Importantly, cardiovascular deaths were independently linked to older subjects, males, non–Hispanic ethnicity, high blood pressure, and cardiovascular morbidity, among other conditions. It is Fiscella's belief that further randomized control trial studies of vitamin D supplementation are warranted for people with low vitamin D levels. The authors concluded that black-white differences in 25 OH Vitamin D levels may contribute to the abundant deaths from cardiovascular disease in black subjects.

5

Kidney Disease

You can maintain healthy functions of the kidneys in many ways. One way is adequate control and management of your blood pressure.

Brief Description of the Kidneys

Although a comprehensive review of kidney function is beyond the scope of this book, the kidneys' functions are vital in meeting the crucial demands of the human body in order to maintain fluid and electrolyte (sodium, potassium, and chloride) balance. The kidneys accomplish this by removing unwanted waste products and extra fluids from the body. In doing so, the kidneys also help regulate blood pressure. The kidneys are found in the abdomen towards the back, with one on each side of the spine (Wedro, 2013). They are two bean-shaped organs that consist of nephrons, an interstitium, and the urine collection system. The kidneys are divided into two regions, the cortex and medulla (Farley & Miller, 1987), otherwise called the outer cortex and inner medulla.

Figure 4 shows normal right and left kidneys.

The functional unit of the kidney is the nephron (Farley & Miller, 1987; Horigan, Rocciccioli, & Trimm, 2012). Approximately one million nephrons are found in each kidney. The nephrons contain many parts, such as the glomerulus, Bowman's capsule, the proximal convoluted tubule, the loop of Henle, the distal convoluted tubule, and the collecting tubule; these take part in the process of forming urine (Farley & Miller, 1987).

Functions of the Kidneys

Our kidneys function to:

1. Filter blood
2. Remove waste products

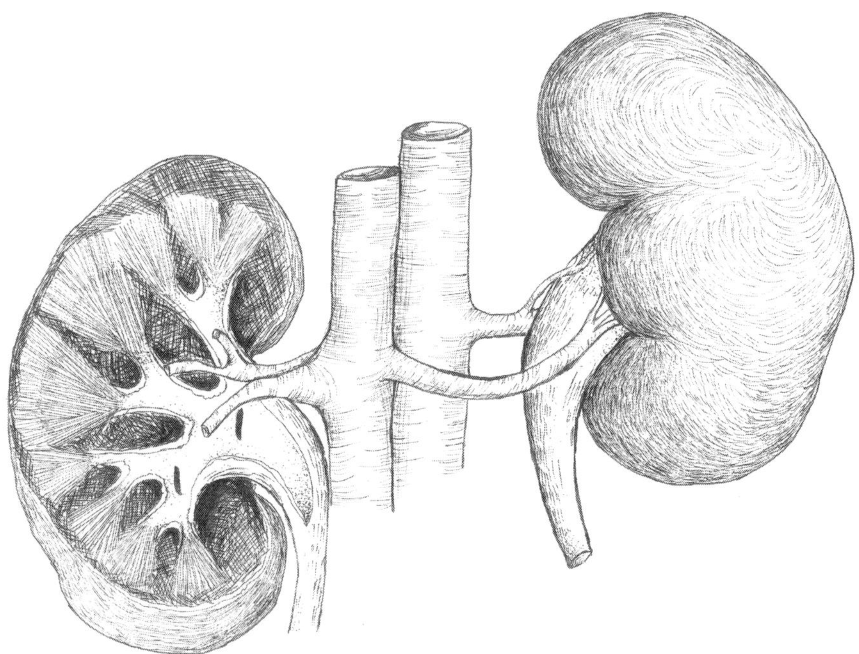

Figure 4. Frontal section of the human left kidney on the left, and the right kidney in a posterior position on the right. The renal veins and arteries are shown extending from each kidney (courtesy Dominique Diedrick).

3. Balance electrolyte levels in the body
4. Control blood pressure
5. Stimulate the production of red blood cells (Wedro, 2015)

Causes of Kidney Disease

Although there are several factors that cause kidney disease, high blood pressure and diabetes are the two main causes (National Kidney Foundation, 2014). The National Kidney Foundation (2014) categorized the risk factors for chronic kidney disease (CKD) as either major risk factors or additional risk factors.

Major Risk Factors

- Diabetes
- Hypertension
- Family history of kidney failure

- Sixty years of age and older
- Autoimmune diseases such as glomerulonephritis

ADDITIONAL RISK FACTORS

- Heart disease
- Obesity
- Smoking
- Kidney stones

Qaseem et al. (2013) have also outlined risk factors for CKD.

MAJOR RISK FACTORS

- Diabetes
- Hypertension
- Cardiovascular disease

OTHER RISK FACTORS

- Older age
- Obesity
- Family history
- African American ethnicity
- Native American or Hispanic ethnicity

The Kidneys: Fluid Balance, Electrolytes, and Waste Products

Without sufficient salt our ancestors would have died of dehydration. In the last century, excessive salt consumption has caused an epidemic of hypertension. The kidneys' primary functions are the same today as those that protected our ancestors in the Paleolithic era from dehydration, a common cause of death. Our ancestors burned more calories and had a greater need for fluids and salt, which was scarce. Although genetic mutations occur over time to help people adapt to change, the industrial revolution, a sedentary lifestyle, and dietary changes, particularly an abundance of salt, occurred too fast for our genes to adapt to these changes. Similar to the ancient mutations that resulted in vitamin D deficiency in dark-skinned individuals today, the genetic changes that protected our ancestors from dehydration now predispose us to hypertension (Goldman, 2015: 91–4).

The kidneys regulate the amount of fluids in the body and filter waste products, such as urea from protein metabolism and uric acid from DNA breakdown.

Blood urea nitrogen (BUN) and creatinine (Cr) are two waste products that can be measured in the blood to help diagnose kidney disease. Whenever blood flows to the kidneys, sensors in the kidneys determine the amount of water to expel as urine and monitor the concentration of electrolytes (Wedro, 2013). Thus, when the nephrons are no longer able to filter wastes and extra fluid, fluid and electrolyte imbalances occur. About 60 percent of the human body is composed of water, and at least one quart is lost each day in urine. Water is needed to flush out the waste products and toxins that result from energy metabolism. Otherwise, these toxins would build up in our bloodstream.

Renin and Blood Pressure

When a person has a sufficient amount of water in the body, his or her urine is more dilute. This makes the urine look clear. Renin, a hormone, controls this regulation. Renin is made in the kidneys and is a necessary part of the fluid and blood pressure regulation systems (Wedro, 2013).

Economic Impact of Kidney Disease in the United States

The treatment of kidney disease in the United States can be costly due to the progression from one stage to the next. According to the National Kidney Foundation (2014), the yearly medical cost for individuals with this condition has increased. For example, from stage 3 to stage 4, the costs increase from $15,000 to $28,000 per year, and reach more than $70,000 in stage 5.

The National Kidney Foundation (2014) documented that not only has the dollar cost of treatment increased, but also people diagnosed with kidney disease visit their physicians an average of 10.3 times a year. Medicare spends almost $30 billion to treat people with kidney failure.

The statistics are staggering for people requiring dialysis treatment and transplants. For example, in 2006 alone, more than 100,000 new patients needed dialysis or transplants, and more than 350,000 people were receiving dialysis.

These figures are high, warranting serious strategies to control and improve health and to decrease the economic burden on the government. Preventive measures, such as education and lifestyle changes, are necessary to increase awareness of kidney disease and to decrease the risk of contributing factors. This is crucial in the United States, and a statewide approach is needed. Emphasis should be targeted to populations who are at greater risk for developing hypertension and diabetes.

Two Major Complications of Chronic Kidney Disease (CKD)

Chronic kidney disease (CKD) is defined as kidney disease that develops over time and lasts longer than 3 months. CKD and end-stage renal diseases (ESRD) are chronic complications caused by hypertension, diabetes, drug toxicity, infections, autoimmune kidney diseases and other conditions. ESRD is the final stage of CKD, and the incidence and prevalence is increasing (Horigan et al., 2012). Harjutsalo and Groop (2014) estimate that in 2013, 382 million people had diabetes. This number is predicted to increase to 592 million by 2035. Harjutsalo and Groop (2014) believe that due to the rising rates of type 1 and type 2 diabetes, the number of people with severe complications (for example, diabetic kidney disease) is also rising. Moreover, 30 to 45 percent of diabetics are likely to end up with ESRD.

Hemodialysis or peritoneal dialysis treatment is required to replace kidney function when CKD complications progress to renal failure (Horigan et al., 2012). Hemodialysis is a medical procedure used to remove wastes and extra fluid from an individual's blood when the kidneys have failed.

Chronic Kidney Disease and Its Prevalence

Studies show that several factors contribute to the prevalence of CKD. For instance, James, Hemmelgarn and Tonelli (2010) reported that the aging population and the increasing global prevalence of diabetes and other chronic noncommunicable diseases have caused a worldwide increase in the prevalence of kidney disease and kidney failure.

Consistent with Inker, Coresh, Levey, Tonelli and Muntner (2011), they also reported that this condition is a major public health problem worldwide, with the effects being an increased prevalence of kidney failure and poor outcome. They also pointed out that the prevalence of CKD in U.S. adults is estimated to be 11.5 percent.

Although the prevalence of CKD has been estimated in many developed countries, its prevalence is not known in developing countries because the standard definition of CKD uses the Modification of Diet in Renal Disease study equation, which is based on the glomerular filtration rate (GFR). The approximate prevalence of CKD in adults is 2.5 to 11 percent across Europe, Asia, North America, and Australia, if the definition of CKD is based on GFRs of less than 60 mL/min/1.73 m^2 (James et al., 2010).

The glomerular filtration rate (GFR) laboratory test, which is also called the estimated GFR or eGFR, is a calculation based on the serum creatinine level, age and race (African American or non-African American). The GFR is used to screen for and detect early kidney damage, to help diagnose CKD, and to monitor kidney status.

Other tests used to measure kidney function include the urine albumin (microalbumin) level and the serum albumin/creatinine ratio (ACR), which is used to screen people with chronic conditions, such as diabetes and hypertension, which put them at an increased risk of developing kidney disease. Increased levels of albumin in the urine may indicate kidney damage.

In the United States, CKD, when it is defined solely on the GFR of less than 60 mL/min/1.73 m,^{2} is over 200-fold more prevalent than kidney failure for those being treated with renal therapy (James et al., 2010). For patients age 65 years and older that have met the criteria for CKD, it is unclear whether their decrease in GFR is related to this condition, or if it is due to the aging process.

Earlier findings from the U.S. Third National Health and Nutritional Examination Survey (obtained from the 1988–1994 database) indicated that the use of the eGFR threshold of 60 mL/min/1.73 m^2 may not benefit people from minority groups (Ibrahim, Wang, Ishani, Collins, & Foley, 2008). Ibrahim et al. indicate that this is because certain metabolic abnormalities often seen in black individuals, primarily an elevated serum uric acid level, high blood pressure, anemia, and increased serum phosphorus, are more prevalent in individuals with higher eGFR values, compared to their white counterparts. It is also documented that the cardiovascular burden, such as illnesses and death, is more pronounced in African Americans in the United States.

Peralta, Weekley, Li and Shlipak (2013) reported that the recommended guidelines established by the Joint National Committee on Prevention, Detection, Evaluation, and Treatment of High Blood Pressure being used to screen persons for CKD may neglect to include some high-risk groups.

The cystatin C blood test, which was formerly known as gamma trace, post-gamma-globulin or neuroendocrine basic polypeptide and is primarily used in research rather than the clinical laboratory, is rarely used as a biomarker of kidney disease and more commonly as a measure of cardiovascular status. Peralta et al. (2013) sugested that the inclusion of cystatin C in screening strategies may be of benefit in detecting people with occult CKD and in the long run may have an effect on their outcomes. They report that this is especially so for individuals with hypertension because screening is presently based on creatinine-derived eGFR used in conjunction with urinalysis tests to screen for protein. However, used with sensitive tests for urine microalbumin, the eGFR is able to detect early kidney disease . Early detection of CKD may help to decrease death rates, especially in the United States, where more than 90,000 Americans die each year from kidney disease (National Kidney Foundation, 2014).

Prevalence of End-Stage Renal Disease

In the United States, 20 million people age 20 years and older have ESRD, and the incidence of this condition is almost four times greater in African Americans than in whites (Stewart, 2013). The incidence of ESRD is also prevalent in other populations, such as Hispanics. Within the Hispanic population, ESRD is frequently attributed to diabetes. Frankenfield, Rocco, Roman and McClellan (2003) stated that the Hispanic population is increasing rapidly, and the rates of diabetes mellitus and hypertension in Hispanics are also high. The authors predict that the treatment percentage of people with ESRD in this specific group will increase significantly in years to come.

Qaseem, Hopkins, Sweet, Starkey and Shekelle (2013) report that CVD, fractures and bone loss, infections, cognitive impairments, and frailty are associated with individuals diagnosed with stages 1 through 3 CKD. They report that even though these individuals are being treated for the associated conditions and complications (hypertension, diabetes, and cardiovascular disease, for example), it is important for clinicians to screen, monitor and treat persons in these stages for specific signs and symptoms related to CKD. These methods are outlined in the American College of Physicians guidelines. Qaseem et al. (2013) emphasized the need for clinicians to target adults for screening and adults with stages 1 through 3 CKD for treatment.

Kidney Disease and Hypertension

There is also a high prevalence of kidney disease in people with hypertension (Peralta et al., 2013), and from the start of the nineteenth century it has been noted that "patients with kidney disease suffer from hypertension" (Ritz, 2007, p. 371).

Yet, there are several potential causes of CKD, and the frequency varies between different populations (James et al., 2010, p. 1297). For instance, in developed countries, age, hypertension, diabetes, smoking, increased BMI, and cardiovascular disease history are consistently linked to this condition.

It is also well documented that people with hypertension are at risk for developing CKD, which can progress to end-stage renal disease (Norris et al., 2008). The literature points to specific groups of people in the population that are mostly affected. For example, Norris et al. (2008) state that minorities are disproportionately at risk for the burdens of ESRD, possibly because of the severity of their hypertension, which is greater, and the prevalence of their hypertension, which is higher.

The incidence of ESRD is also reported to be an alarming 1.5 to 4 times higher in minorities in the United States compared to their white counterparts (Norris et al., 2008). Norris et al. (2008) believe that this rate implies a distinct difference in the progression of CKD in minority groups. Martins, Agodoa and Norris (2012) report that disparity is notable in minority groups compared to whites; diabetes and hypertension rates are higher in blacks, they develop these conditions earlier, their diseases are poorly controlled, and complications, such as CKD, occur at higher rates in this group.

This suggests that "the higher rate of hypertension and the lower rate of blood pressure control in African Americans with CKD may contribute to the more rapid progression of CKD to end-stage renal disease" (Martins et al., 2012, p. 2). However, the prevalence of CKD is growing most rapidly in people 60 years and older (National Kidney and Urologic Diseases Information Clearinghouse, 2012).

There is a rising incidence of CKD in the United States, and the costs to treat people with CKD and ESRD have also increased. For example, there was an increase of 10 percent in the cost of treatment for adults in the United States with stages 1 through 4 CKD from 1988 to 1994, and an increase of 13 percent from 1999 to 2004. It cost the U.S. government $23 billion to treat people with ESRD in 2006. Within the same year, the overall cost to treat people with CKD was $49 billion (Appel et al., 2010). Appel et al. (2010) report that in the United States, hypertension burden is the cause of approximately 30 percent of all cases of ESRD and CKD.

James et al. (2010) suggest that the ultimate management strategy would be to treat people with hypertension in order to slow the progress of CKD and decrease cardiovascular risk in those without diabetic CKD. James et al. (2010) believe that this sort of management is required because with an increase in blood pressure to 130/80 mm Hg, individuals are at increased risk of CKD progression and kidney failure. Consistent with Yamount et al. (2014), they stated that even though aggressive treatment measures for several risk factors are needed for decreasing death and improving kidney disease, the management of hypertension is most important.

Does Weight Play a Role in the Development of Chronic Kidney Disease?

Studies suggests that weight is another risk factor for developing CKD, particularly in minorities, such as African Americans. A longitudinal study of

3,430 African American men and women between 21 to 94 years of age who resided in the tri-county area of Jackson, Mississippi, was conducted by Bruce et al. (2013). The study participants' mean age was 54, 63.7 percent were women, and 54.8 percent were married. The researchers exploited data from the baseline examination of the Jackson Heart Study to determine participants' CKD status. This study is believed to be one of the largest single-site cohort studies of CVD in African Americans.

For this study, CKD was defined as the presence of albuminuria, or decreased estimated glomerular filtration rate (eGFR) that was less than 60 mL/min/1.73 m.[2] It is important to note that this criterion for defining CKD was broader, compared to other studies that defined CKD only on baseline eGFR. Weight status was measured using four categories, based on BMI.

The findings of the study showed that the rate of CKD was 20 percent. Eighty-five percent of the participants were classified as overweight or obese. Twenty-six percent had BMIs over 35. More significantly, BMIs more than or equal to 35 signified a major risk factor for men, but not for women. This result was noted after an adjustment of demographic, clinical, and socioeconomic variables. Nevertheless, the prevalence of CKD risk factors was reported to be high.

The percentages of CKD for individuals with different health conditions varied. For instance, 62 percent had hypertension, 31 percent had hypercholesterolemia, 18 percent had diabetes, 10 percent had CVD, and 7 percent had hypertriglyceridemia (an elevated serum triglyceride level). Group differences that looked at age, access to health care, marital status, income levels, and hypercholesterolemia were modest and significant, yet not clinically relevant. However, when compared to the group-specific results that looked at major risk factors for CKD and CKD measures, it showed that subjects who were obese had a larger percentage of diabetes, hypertension, albuminuria, and decreased eGFR.

Subjects in the "women only" models showed that being overweight, class I obesity, and class II obesity were not condition risks for CKD when compared to women who were of normal weight. However, weight status was significant in the "men only" model. Men who were in the heaviest weight category were twice as likely to have CKD, compared to men of normal weight. Interestingly, CVD was associated with CKD for women and men. For those classified as normal weight and both class II obese women and men with CVD risks, risks for developing CKD were higher (Bruce et al., 2013).

According to Bruce et al. (2013), their study highlighted the need for further studies to look at the relationship between obesity and CKD in African American people. A previous study cited by Bruce et al. (2013) had shown contrasting findings, showing that waist to hip ratio, and not BMI, had been linked to CKD. The contrasts between these studies possibly resulted from differences in study participants' characteristics. The earlier study cohort, according to these authors, was larger and more heterogeneous in racial profile, and the prevalence of baseline risk factors such as hypertension, diabetes, and CVD was lower.

Bruce et al.'s (2013) findings demonstrated the sex-specific patterns of weight, CKD, and their relation among African Americans. They stated that further studies need to be completed, and that these studies should examine the relationship between excess weight, health outcomes, and kidney disease in African American people.

Szomba (2012) examined the effects of obesity on conditions associated with CKD and reported that adult subjects with BMIs higher than 35 kg/m^2 have a sevenfold increased chance of diabetes and hypertension diagnoses. This author states that hypertension and diabetes "are the most common causes of CKD" (p. 132); a recent U.S. study reported that 24.2 percent of kidney disease in men and 33 percent in women is believed to be caused from being overweight and obesity. Szomba (2012) states that even though some of the reported effects were mediated by hypertension and diabetes, having more body weight and fat might play a role in the rate and development of CKD.

Szomba (2012) also reported another study of a population in Cuba that looked at the prevalence of obesity and overweight conditions, and whether these were associated with CKD, hypertension, diabetes, and the risk factors for the aforementioned conditions.

Of the participants more than 20 years of age, 31 percent were overweight, 13.4 percent of which were characterized as obese; 21.2 percent of the overweight participants had markers that were positive for kidney damage; and 32.7 percent of obese subjects had a microalbuminuria value that had increased with weight increase. The prevalence of hypertension was 31.5 percent in overweight persons and 51.9 percent in obese persons. Interestingly, the more weight subjects gained, their diabetes risk increased, and the prevalence almost tripled to 11.3 percent in those who were obese.

In comparison, for subjects under the age of 20, the prevalence of obesity was 3.2 percent. Albuminuria was present in 38 percent of the obese individuals and only 3 percent in those who were not obese, while diabetes was prevalent in 9.5 percent of the obese people and only 1.1 percent in nonobese.

This suggests that more longitudinal research studies are needed in both younger and older age categories for people of various ethnic backgrounds in North American and other developing countries. The findings will help to determine whether increased weight status plays such a significant role in CKD development and progression, because it is well documented that diabetes and hypertension are the main reasons for CKD. These findings will also help in implementing early preventive measures within communities to address those at risk for kidney disease.

Left Ventricular Hypertrophy and Hypertensive Chronic Kidney Disease

Peterson et al. (2013) studied the relationship between left ventricular hypertrophy (LVH) and diastolic dysfunction and adverse outcomes in 578 African Americans who had hypertensive CKD to determine whether there was an association with CVD and renal outcomes. This African American Study of Kidney Disease observational hypertensive cohort study was an extension of a trial that examined African Americans with nondiabetic hypertensive kidney disease that had not reached ESRD.

Peterson et al. (2013) states that other studies have evaluated whites of European background and found LVH (left ventricular hypertrophy) to be linked to coronary artery disease and increased illnesses and death. But although it has been reported by Peterson et al. (2013) that the prevalence of LVH is greater in African Americans than in their white counterparts, that those with CKD are more likely to experience adverse outcomes, and that this population with hypertension is at increased risk for CKD, epidemiological studies have not addressed this group as they should.

To address this, the researchers studied whether there were any adverse outcomes in this group with hypertensive CKD. Subjects were 691 African Americans followed for a five-year period. Baseline echocardiograms were repeated at 24- and 48-month follow-up visits. Measurements for levels of ambulatory blood pressure, albumin, and creatinine were also taken. Outcomes were assessed and defined, such as main CVD composite, main renal composite, and heart failure alone, which was defined as the first hospital admission or death from an episode of heart failure.

The study showed that the echocardiographically (ECG) defined LVH was a strong predictor of heart failure and other CVD outcomes, even when adjustments for several clinical factors such as gender, sex, baseline eGFR, and adjustment of diastolic dysfunction were made. Greater LV mass index had a significant association with higher chance of CVD risk outcomes. Also, certain measures of diastolic function had an association with later heart failure. However, there was no independent association with renal outcomes in these participants.

Peterson et al. (2013) demonstrated that shortened deceleration time is associated with hospitalization in the future, and lower E/A ratios, a marker of diastolic dysfunction, are also associated with heart failure in the future. They believed that echocardiographic risk factors may help to recognize CKD high-risk individuals for aggressive therapy interventions.

It is important to note that these participants were part of a younger age group. Nevertheless, Peterson et al. (2013) concluded that their study raised the importance of echocardiography in identifying individuals with hypertensive CKD who may be at risk for heart failure and other cardiovascular events. They also pointed to the need for further studies to examine echocardiographic parameters, because the findings may help reduce health-adverse events in this vulnerable population.

Diabetic Kidney Disease and Blood Pressure

Harjutsalo and Groop (2014) believe there is a correlation between the kidneys and blood pressure because kidney disease results in an increase in blood pressure. When blood pressure increases, it speeds up the loss of kidney function. The authors stated that the main treatment and preventive measures for diabetic kidney disease are to block the renin-angiotensin system (RAS) with the use of medications that also work to lower blood pressure. They further linked this success to other studies, such as the Reduction in Endpoints in Noninsulin-Dependent Diabetes Mellitus with Angiotensin II Antagonist Losartan study and the Irbesartan Diabetic Nephropathy Trial.

These studies had demonstrated a delay in diabetic kidney disease when blood pressure was effectively controlled and RAS blockaded, which is consistent with Yamout et al. (2014), a study pointing to the benefits of renin-angiotensin-aldosterone system (RAAS) blockade in subjects with advanced stage 3 CKD whose levels of proteinuria are above 500 mg/day.

Definition of Chronic Kidney Disease

Peralta et al. (2013) define CKD "as an estimated glomerular filtration rate (eGFR) of less than 60 mL/min/1.73 m^2 or the presence of albuminuria (albumin-to-creatinine ratio in urine greater than 30 mg/g)" (p. 1196). Martins et al. (2012), however, defined CKD based on the 2002 National Kidney Foundation's definition. They stated that one of the definitions of CKD is 3 or more months of kidney damage where structural or functional abnormalities are seen in the kidney and where there either is or isn't a decrease in the GFR. This is shown in pathologic abnormalities or markers of kidney damage in combination with abnormalities in formation of blood or urine, such as proteinuria, or abnormalities in imaging tests. The other definition, they state, of CKD is GFR less than 60mL/min/1.73 m^2 for 3 months or more, with or without kidney damage.

The Five Stages of Chronic Kidney Disease and Their Detection

Martin et al. (2012) divided CKD into five progressive stages based on GFR. According to these authors, in stage 1 there is kidney damage with normal or increased GFR (GFR greater than 90 mL/min/1.73 m^2). In stage 2, there is notable kidney damage and mildly decreased GFR (60–89 mL/min/1.73 m^2). Stage 3 patients have a moderately decreased GFR (30–59 mL/min/1.73 m^2). In stage 4, GFR is severely decreased (15–29 mL/min/1.73 m^2). Lastly, in stage 5 the kidneys fail and GFR is less than 15 mL/min/1.73 m,[2] and dialysis is necessary.

The authors point to notable early detection in the stages of kidney disease in individuals, based on the definition of CKD, which consists of markers (for example, albuminuria) that show kidney damage "when estimated GFR may be still within normal limits" (Martins et al., 2012, p. 2).

Qaseem et al. (2013) stated that although CKD has been defined traditionally as five stages based on GFR, additional categories are needed to define CKD severity *in combination* with these five stages of GFR.

According to Qaseem et al. (2013), CKD stages 1–3 are known as the early stages, where people with them show no symptoms. As such, laboratory tests or imaging are used to diagnose CKD. Qaseem et al. (2013) included three categories of albuminuria levels in their study to define the severity of CKD. This definition was based on the 2013 Kidney Disease Improving Global Outcomes revision of CKD staging.

Qaseen et al. (2013) stated that an estimated 22.4 million adults in the United States have stage 1–3 CKD, and that the prevalence is rising even more for stage 3 CKD. The authors also discovered that almost half of the people with this condition have stage 1 or 2 CKD, and one-third of those have higher albuminuria, whereas two-thirds have normal albuminuria. The occurrence of CKD is slightly higher in women, at 12.6 percent, compared to men, at 9.7 percent.

Modalities for Kidney Failure—Brief Statistics

Studies have pointed to the need for donor kidneys and encouraged living donor kidney transplantation (Nogueira et al., 2009). In addition to the grave need for live kidney donors, individuals with renal decline will continue to require dialysis treatment to sustain their lives; most of these individuals are on the waiting list for suitable kidney transplants. The National Kidney Foundation (2014) stated that 120,000 Americans are waiting for lifesaving organ transplants. Of these individuals, 99,000 require a kidney. But despite these large numbers, fewer than 17,000 of these individuals receive a kidney in a given year (National Kidney Foundation, 2014).

Hypertension and Kidney Disease

Research has continually shown that people with hypertension and diabetes are at greater risk for kidney failure. As such, many of these individuals will require dialysis treatment until kidneys from suitable donors are available for transplantation.

Uncontrolled blood pressure may play a role in kidney damage. This may be due to the low percentage of hypertensive individuals in the United States who have their blood pressure under control. Of the estimated 65 million Americans with hypertension, only one-third of these individuals have their blood pressure under control (Gross, Anderson, Busby, Frith, & Panco, 2013). In African American people, 72 percent do not have their blood pressure controlled within normal ranges (Peters, Aroian, & Flack, 2006). The National Kidney Foundation (2014) stated that in the United States, a black person's likelihood of experiencing kidney failure is three times higher than whites, and for Hispanics the likelihood is one and a half times greater. Similarly, African Americans receive hemodialysis treatment at rates four times greater than whites. The incidence rate for ESRD is also higher in African Americans than in whites, almost four times higher (Stewart, 2013).

Further, Cozier et al. (2006) stated that illness prevalence, for example, that of CVD or ESRD, is higher in black women in the United States, and these conditions are believed to be hypertension related. Moreover, in black women the rate of hypertension is two to three times higher than in white women, and the age-specific rate for black women is believed to be similar to those white women in the next age decade.

Uncontrolled Blood Pressure and Chronic Kidney Disease

Studies show that uncontrolled blood pressure gives rise to complications, such as CKD, which can progress to ESRD. For example, Peterson et al. (2013) reported that African American people at risk for hypertension are also at greater risk for the development of CKD, and their risk of adverse events is also higher. According to Bruce et al. (2013), these individuals tend to need transplantation and dialysis at younger ages, and the incidence of ESRD is higher with every 10 years of life, in comparison to other racial or ethnic groups.

Bruce et al. (2013) further stated that "kidney disease is one of the most pressing yet underemphasized issues in American public health" (p. 710) and that one in eight people greater than 20 years of age is affected with a form of CKD. More than 20 million U.S. adults are at risk for kidney failure or ESRD, and possibly other complications due to kidney disease.

Autoimmune Diseases and Chronic Kidney Disease

Autoimmune diseases may be systemic, affecting multiple organs and systems. For example, in systemic lupus erythematosus (SLE), the disease process can target the heart, lungs, kidneys (lupus nephritis) and other organs. Autoimmune diseases may also be organ specific, targeting one organ, for instance the kidneys in Goodpasture's syndrome. Glomerulonephritis, one of the most common autoimmune kidney disorders, may occur in patients with SLE or it may develop as an organ-specific disease.

The prevalence of autoimmune kidney disease varies by race. For instance 40 percent of cases of SLE are seen in African Americans, which is another reason for higher incidences of CKD in this population. Thirty-eight percent of cases are seen in whites, 15 percent of cases in Hispanics, 5 percent in Asians, and 2 percent in Native Americans. Complications of SLE resulting in death are most likely to occur in Native Americans, and least likely to occur in Hispanics and Asians (Preidt, 2015).

In IgA nephropathy, another autoimmune kidney disease, is a type of glomerulonephritis. In the United States, Canada, and the United Kingdom, IgA nephropathy accounts for 2–10 percent of glomerular kidney diseases, but in Japan, it accounts for 18–40 percent of cases. IgA nephropathy often begins in older children or young adults in their 20s and 30s. The disease occurs more often in males, rarely occurs in blacks and tends to run in families, which suggests that genetics play a part in who develops it. About 30–40 percent of individuals with this disorder develop ESRD (Kugler, 2016).

Other autoimmune diseases that can affect the kidneys include type 1 diabetes; pulmonary-renal syndrome; gluten sensitivity and celiac disease; Crohn's disease; inflammatory bowel disease (IBD); interstitial nephritis; ANCA associated vasculitis; Henoch-Schönlein purpura; Wegener's granulomatosis; polyarteritis nodosa (PAN); and sarcoidosis.

End-Stage Renal Disease Treatment in the United States

Dialysis is a life-support treatment that uses a special machine to filter harmful wastes, salt, and excess fluid from your blood, performing the kidney's normal functions in patients with kidney disease. Lok and Foley (2013) reported that over the past 10 years, more than one million North Americans started dialysis, and in 2010 alone the ESRD program in the United States treated 593,086 persons. Of this amount, 383,992 had hemodialysis treatment, "(64.7 percent of all patients with ESRD or 92.8 percent of all dialysis patients)" (Lok & Foley, 2013, p. 1213). The combined incidence was 348 individuals with ESRD per million people, to 105,923 hemodialysis patients, whereas the prevalence was 1,752 per million people, which equals 383,992 hemodialysis patients. Lok and Foley (2013) explained that even though the yearly incidence of new patients was stable, in 2010 the prevalence had increased 49.0 percent since 2000. The National Kidney Foundation (2014) reported that almost 430,000 persons in America are receiving dialysis treatment and approximately 185,000 people are living with a functional kidney that they acquired through transplant.

These high statistics illustrate the need for drastic measures to effectively control high blood pressure and diabetes in the American population. The aim is to institute preventive interventions in every state, increase awareness of high blood pressure, and educate the public about these chronic conditions and their consequences. This may help to decrease prevalence and incidence rates of chronic kidney disease and subsequently prevent kidney failure. If conditions of hypertension are detected early, interventions may result in improved treatment and possibly improved prognosis in this population.

Peritoneal Dialysis and Hemodialysis

In peritoneal dialysis, extra water and waste products are removed from the patient's body. Blood is cleansed while inside the individual's body (Kidney Foundation of Canada, 2014).

In hemodialysis, blood is withdrawn from the individual's body and filtered by machine; with peritoneal dialysis a machine is not used.

People with ESRD require either hemodialysis (HD) or peritoneal dialysis (PD) treatment to survive. HD and PD were developed at different times in the twentieth century as treatment options for chronic uremic (having waste products from urine in the blood circulation, which is a sign of kidney [renal] disease) patients. HD emerged at the end of the 1960s, thanks to the pioneers who researched and facilitated the process of vascular access to sustain the lives of patients with ESRD, whereas PD was introduced towards the late 1970s (Cancarini, 2004).

Cancarini (2004) stated that although PD is utilized less frequently than HD, PD modalities differ in terms of its penetration among countries and within different parts of the same country. But despite one method being used more frequently and its availability in various locales, Cancarini (2004) believes that comparing these modalities is difficult. This may be because several "factors oppose an adequate balance of the many factors influencing the patient's outcome" (p. S67). For instance, Lameire and Biesen (2004) stated that the survival factor is residual renal function regardless of the method used.

Vascular Access: A Brief History of the Pioneers

According to Lok and Foley (2013), Dr. Nils Alwall initially came up with the idea of maintaining arteriovenous (AV) access patency with the use of a glass cannula in 1948. However, Alwall decided not to proceed with this brilliant idea because of the potential risk of complications, such as infection and clotting.

In 1960, Dr. Belding Scribner and an engineer named Wayne Quinton described the original all–Teflon (polytetrafluoroethylene or PTFE) Quinton-Scribner AV shunt. This AV shunt had a survival rate of 2 months. However, after 2 years, Quinton and Scribner decided to change their original shunt by attaching flexible silicon-rubber tubing. They joined this tubing between the cannulated vessels using Telfon, and it became known as the "silastic-Telfon shunt." This modified device had an increased lifespan device of months and sometimes years. Quinton and Scribner's shunt was a medical advancement, but others were also brainstorming the idea of an extended and viable access.

In 1962, doctors Cimino, Brescia, and Appel created the arteriovenous fistula (AV fistula), which to date is the preferred vascular access for treating hemodialysis patients (Lok & Foley, 2013).

Three Types of Vascular Access

For the purpose of this chapter, only the internal AV fistula is discussed, because it is the preferred vascular access for patients requiring dialysis treatment (Kidney Foundation of Canada, 2010), and the preferred vascular access for HD (Lok & Foley, 2013). The Kidney Foundation of Canada (2010, p. 1) outlines three common access types.

1. Internal arteriovenous fistula
2. Internal arteriovenous graft
3. Central venous catheter, also called central venous "line" or hemodialysis catheter

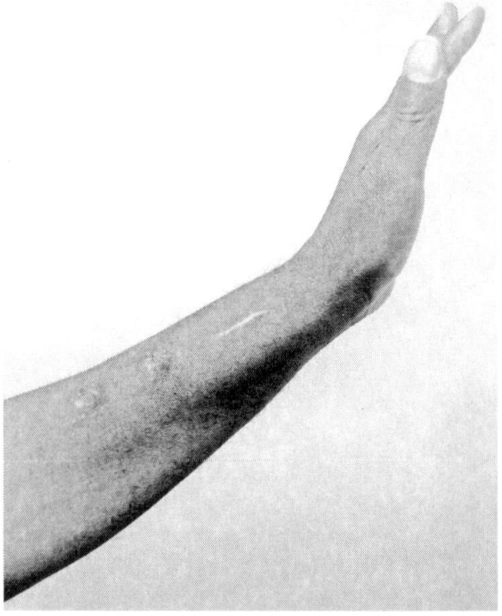

Figure 5. A dialysis patient's arm with the arteriovenous (AV) fistula between the thumb and the needle sites. The AV fistula was surgically created to connect an artery to a vein, where it is accessed for hemodialysis.

Arteriovenous Fistula

AV fistula is an abnormal connection or passageway between an artery and a vein. Figure 5 depicts an AV fistula and needle sites.

An AV fistula can be congenital or surgically created for people requiring dialysis treatment, or it can be a pathologic process resulting from some trauma or erosion of an arterial aneurysm.

When a person needs hemodialysis, a connection to the blood vessels is required to remove wastes and extra fluid from the blood. To achieve this, the doctor, after discussion with the patient, will perform minor surgery to create a fistula. An AV fistula for hemodialysis treatment is created by joining an artery

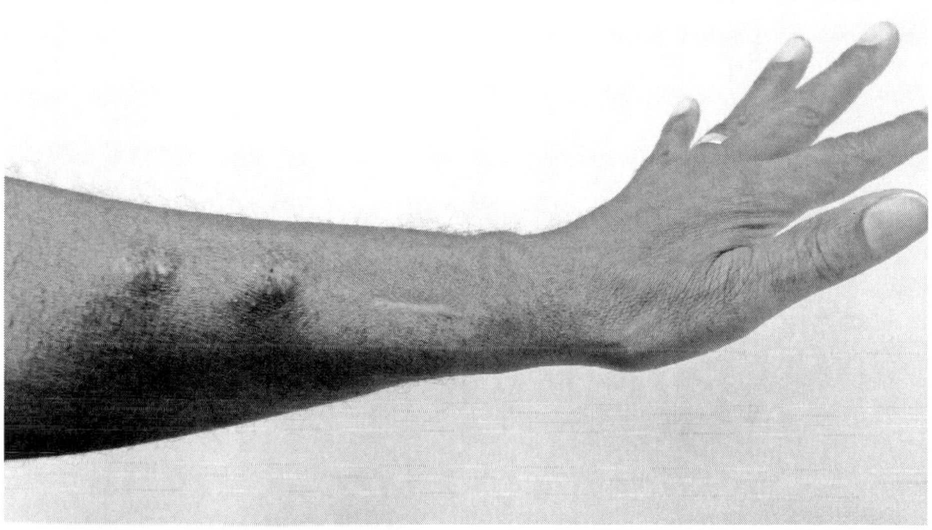

Figure 6. A dialysis patient's arm with a horizontal view of the AV fistula between the thumb and the needle sites. The two needle sites are used for hemodialysis.

to a vein. This provides medical staff quick and efficient access to the patient's blood stream for dialysis (Kidney Foundation of Canada, 2010). Figure 6 shows a horizontal view of an AV fistula and two needle sites.

This access allows the patient's blood to move through flexible tubes to the dialysis machine. The patient's blood is cleansed as it passes through a filter called the dialyzer (National Kidney Foundation, 2006). The AV fistula is the global preference for accessing the blood stream of dialysis patients (National Kidney Foundation, 2006).

It is mandatory that the AV fistula matures before it can be used for hemodialysis treatment, and this "usually takes between four to six weeks" (Kidney Foundation of Canada, 2010, p. 2).

The Kidney Foundation of Canada (2010) outlines the method for utilizing the fistula for dialysis as follows:

> At the dialysis unit, the dialysis nurse will put two needles into the individual's fistula to provide treatment. Once treatment is completed these are removed. The individual will be instructed to apply light pressure for 10 minutes to assist in clotting of blood at needle sites. It is important to follow the instruction directed by the dialysis staff person. If the individual has left the dialysis unit and bleeding starts at the needle sites again, light pressure is applied but for 20 minutes this time. However, if it continues the individual should seek medical attention at an emergency department.

Figure 7 shows a horizontal view of the needle sites.

Advantages of Arteriovenous Fistula

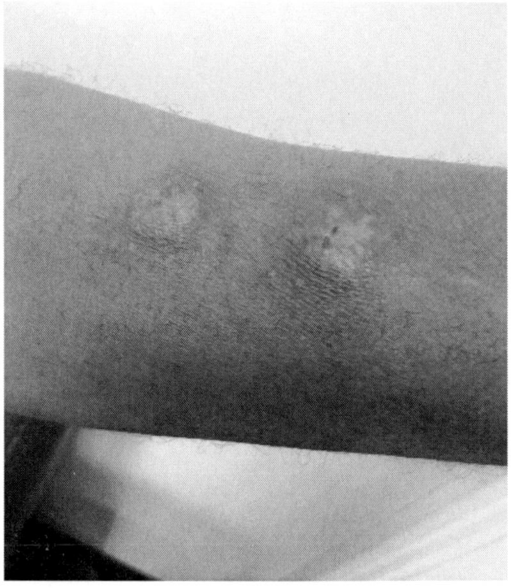

Figure 7. A dialysis patient's arm with two needle sites. The dialysis nurse inserts two needles into the needle sites during hemodialysis. One needle carries the patient's blood from the body to the artificial machine (dialyzer). After the dialyzer filters the blood, the other needle carries the blood back to the patient's body.

- Risk of infection and blood clotting is less
- Risk of the fistula becoming blocked is low
- Blood flow is good after the access site is healed
- Patient can shower post-surgery after the access is healed (National Kidney Foundation, 2006)
- Lasts longer in comparison to AV grafts and central venous catheters (Kidney Foundation of Canada, 2010)

Disadvantages

- Needles are placed in the access site to connect to the dialyzer machine
- Has to mature 1 to 4 months post-surgery before it can be used for dialysis (National Kidney Foundation, 2006)

Maintenance of Arteriovenous Fistula

According to the Kidney Foundation of Canada (2010), patients with an AV fistula must care for it at all times. The patient should check for vibrating sensation by touching the site just above the surgical incision line. The sensation should feel like a "thrill," and it is a sign that the AV fistula is functioning as blood flows through it. It is also necessary to monitor for any changes in color, temperature, tingling or numbness sensations, and swelling, or any form of bleeding from the fistula. This can be done by checking the hand on the side where the AV fistula is situated. If the patient experiences any of these symptoms, the surgeon or nephrology team should be informed. The National Kidney Foundation (2006) has stated that blood should not be taken from the same arm as the one with an AV fistula. Also, blood pressure should be taken and injections given in the arm that does not feature the fistula.

Studies show that even though PD and HD are both dialysis modalities in current use, a patient's long-term outcome, in terms of illnesses and death, differs between these two modalities. Cancarini (2004) discussed previous studies that looked at whether PD could provide patient survival rates similar to those of HD. According to Cancarini (2004), the CANUSA study done on PD patients in the United States reported a twofold increase in the risk of death. The study findings were compared to PD patients treated in Canada. The data for Canadian results were outlined in the Canadian Organ Replacement Register. It showed that only patients who were diabetic and over 65 years of age showed death risks similar for those who received PD and HD; however, PD diabetic and nondiabetic patients of a younger age had risk of death rates significantly lower.

But according to Cancarini (2004), the incident cohort study of USRDS patients from 1995 to 1997 found that the risk of death was similar for diabetic PD and HD patients in model one while in model two, PD diabetic patient risk of death was higher. Nevertheless, the risk of death had declined in patients who were not diabetic.

In terms of morbidity (illnesses), Cancarini (2004) further stated that patients receiving PD needed longer hospital stays than those receiving HD, even though the patient admission rate was similar for both modalities. Cancarini (2004) emphasized that two study findings did not show a significant difference between PD and HD, whereas some studies showed differences—some demonstrated better results for those patients on PD, while others showed the opposite.

The health condition of the individual may be a factor for persons on PD. For example, Cancarini (2004) reported that anemia and lower glomerular filtration rate (GFR) are associated with poorer quality of life. The author further reported that ischemic heart disease is a frequent complication in patients on dialysis, and although some studies suggest that patients with chronic heart failure should use PD, others disagree. This is because in patients with chronic heart failure, risk of death is higher with PD compared to HD patients—1.30 in diabetics and 1.24 in nondiabetics.

Cancarini (2004) concluded that "technique survival is definitely worse in PD" (p. S69) and "sclerosing encapsulating peritonitis is one of the more dangerous changes in peritoneal membrane" (p. S69).

Live Kidney Donors and African Americans

Although live kidney donors are encouraged, studies show that long-term health effects, such as renal complications resulting from unilateral nephrectomy done on healthy people, are concerning. This is especially so for African Americans. The Nogueira et al. (2009) study sought African American Living Kidney Donors (AALKDs) who had donated at the University of Maryland Medical Center between March 1, 1996, and February 28, 2002. One hundred seven donors were invited for follow-up health evaluation. The purpose of the study was to describe AALKD renal outcomes several years after they donated by comparing AALKDs with non–African American donors.

For this study, hypertension was defined and renal function was estimated using five different equations. One equation was the abbreviated Modification of Diet in Renal Disease (MDRD) equation estimated glomerular filtration rate, or eGFR(MDRD) (Nogueira et al., 2009, p. 1372). The prevalence of microalbuminuria was 16 percent, while 16 people (41 percent) had hypertension at follow-up. These people were compared to non-donor African Americans. It was also revealed that eGFR was less than 60 mL/min/1.73 m,[2] and absolute and relative loss of eGFR was a lot higher in AALKDs who were obese, compared to those who were not. The authors believe that the risk factors for CKD may be an issue in live kidney donors. Also, the high rate of hypertension observed in AALKDs is concerning because none of the study participants had hypertension at the start of the study. They also believe that "hypertension may be more nephrotoxic in African Americans, given those individuals with one kidney have less renal reserve" (p. 1376). Their findings raised the need for further studies, which would involve counseling and guidance in the selection process of AALKDs. The authors also strongly believe that AALKDs should be monitored for hypertension and CKD.

Statistics show that there are a large number of individuals awaiting suitable kidney donors. But according to Gill, Rose, Pereira and Torelli (2007), sometimes the analyzed results are shown for those who receive kidney transplantation. Gill et al. (2007) believed that the transplant process should include the survival of study subjects on the wait list and those with failed kidney transplants. They conducted a study to investigate the death rates during the continuum of wait list to transplantation and after allograft failure. This was carried out among adult patients with ESRD in the United States between 1996 and 2003. Most of the study participants were male whites under 50 years of age. The authors described the death rates while study subjects were going through the transplant experience from wait list to transplantation and back to receiving dialysis after transplant had failed. It is important to note that more participants were on the wait list in recent years, while most were activated to the wait list within a year after they started dialysis treatment. For 36 percent of the participants, diabetes was the reason for ESRD.

The findings demonstrated that death rates gradually increased during the wait list period and increased quickly among diabetic participants. There was an increase in death rates when wait time for transplantation increased. When people were removed from the wait list, death rates were reported to be higher. Of most interest, CVD was the main cause of death during the wait list time frame.

However, death rates were shown to be greater during the peri-transplant period. Also, more deaths were noted when patients returned to dialysis after their allograft had failed. Nevertheless, death rates were lower in those with an allograft that was functional, and there was no increase in death rates during three years of observation. It was also shown that the longer the period of time those patients had to undergo dialysis before receiving transplantation, the higher the death rates.

The findings also revealed that risk of death increased for people who had higher residual renal function and had returned to dialysis after their allograft had failed. It is worthwhile to note that the duration of allograft survival had no connection with survival after transplant had failed.

The findings suggest the importance of careful monitoring of individuals from the initial assessment for kidney transplant, the entire period of the dialysis treatment process, and beyond. These measures will help to identify those at risk for death and implement meaningful strategies to decrease death rates, thus improving the quality of health for people with ESRD.

6

Stroke and Cerebrovascular Disease

People with high blood pressure can reduce the risk of stroke and decrease their chances of disabilities from stroke if they religiously take their blood pressure medication and carry out daily, meaningful, healthy lifestyle habits.

This chapter provides a literature review on cerebrovascular disease and stroke. It includes a discussion of stroke's relation to hypertension, disability from stroke, prevalence of stroke, types of stroke, and mortality (deaths) and morbidity (illnesses). Preventive measures, such as health and lifestyle behavioral changes, are also covered.

Cerebrovascular disease refers to a group of conditions, including aneurysms, which affect the circulation of blood to the brain, causing limited or no blood flow to affected areas of the brain. One of the most common causes of cerebrovascular disease is atherosclerosis. Stroke occurs as a cerebrovascular accident or CVA.

A body of research has continually documented that hypertension is a major risk factor not only for heart disease and kidney disease but also for stroke. Hypertension is also an important risk factor that is modifiable for primary prevention of ischemic and hemorrhagic stroke (Mackenzie et al., 2013).

Feng, Pang and Beard (2104) stated that "hypertension is the most and strongest modifiable risk factor for stroke" (p. 1); worldwide, the ratio of adult people with hypertension is one in three, which contributes to 51 percent of all deaths due to stroke (Feng et al., 2014). It is well known that people with elevated blood pressure are at risk of stroke (Hatori et al., 2014). Given the high prevalence of hypertension and documented uncontrolled hypertension, especially in the U.S. population, it is a priority that the disease be adequately controlled and managed.

Stroke Mortality Reduction in the United States

According to Go et al. (2014), in the United States alone, on an average, someone suffers a stroke every 40 seconds. Additionally, someone dies from a stroke almost every 4 minutes. This statistic is grave. Nonetheless, Go et al. (2014) stated that the reduction in stroke deaths over the past 10 years and other factors, such as population health improvements in males and females of all ages and races, has had an impact on the decrease in stroke incidence and fatality rates. Most importantly, the efforts to control hypertension, which were introduced in the 1970s, seem to be "the most substantial influence on the accelerated decline in stroke mortality, with lower blood pressure distributions in the population" (p. 401), as well as programs to control diabetes mellitus and high cholesterol, and reduce smoking. The various hypertension treatments all have played a role in lowering stroke deaths.

The Morbidity and Mortality Weekly Report (MMWR, 2013) reported that the fourth leading cause of long-term disability in the United States is stroke, and high blood pressure is the single most important risk factor for this condition. Not only does disability from stroke affect people in the United States, but stroke is the leading cause of serious long-term disability, as well as the second-highest reason for death globally (Zhong et al., 2014). Consistent with Zhong (2014) and (Feng et al., 2014), they also reported that one of the leading causes of death and disability in adults around the world is stroke.

Risk Factors for Stroke

There are many risk factors for stroke and some stroke risk factors are controllable while others are not. However, "hypertension is the most important single risk factor for stroke and its control is essential to reducing death from stroke" (MMWR, 2013, p. 721). According to McDonnell et al. (2013), physical inactivity is the second leading risk factor. The literature points to other identified risk factors, but the risk factors mentioned are those for ischemic stroke in people 15 to 49 years of age. For example, dyslipidemia is the most common one (60 percent), followed by smoking (44 percent), and arterial hypertension (39 percent) "with accumulation in men and increasing age" (von Sarnowski et al., 2013, p. 120). Another risk factor for stroke is sickle cell disease. While all sickle cell genotypes are associated with increased risk, patients with sickle cell anemia are at highest risk with a prevalence of 4.01 percent (Ohene-Frempong et al., 1998).

Alkadry, Bhandari and Blessett (2011) have outlined both nonmodifiable risk factors and modifiable risk factors for stroke. According to the authors, nonmodifiable stroke risk factors are the following.

- Race
- Age
- Family history
- Previous Stroke

Modifiable risk factors are the following.

- Hypertension
- Smoking
- Obesity
- Cholesterol
- Diabetes
- Physical inactivity
- Use of alcohol

If death rates and disability from stroke are to be minimized or prevented, people with hypertension must optimize lifestyle measures to control their blood pressure. Stroke can affect young and older people of different ethnic backgrounds. Moreover, people with risk factors for stroke can experience a stroke event. But, their risk will increase if they have high blood pressure.

Possible Cause of Stroke

Zhong et al. (2014) stated that there is a positive association between homocysteine (Hcy), which is a sulphur-containing amino acid associated with abnormal blood clotting, and stroke incidence. For example, a 5 umol/ 1 Hcy rise results in a 59 percent increase in the risk of stroke whereas, a 3 umol /1 Hcy decrease results in a 24 percent reduction in the risk of stroke. High homocysteine levels are associated with hypercoagulation syndromes and these disorders, which are often autoimmune (for instance antiphospholipid syndrome), may affect both men and women. These conditions often emerge in young adults and are the leading cause of strokes and recurrent miscarriages in young women.

How Does Stroke Happen?

Alkadry et al. (2011) state that a stroke happens when the blood supply to the individual brain cells is quickly interrupted, which results in immediate death of some brain cells. Concurrently, damage is done to other brain cells in the region of the injury.

Prevalence of Stroke

Mitka (2011) stated that people in the United States who have implemented healthier lifestyle choices may have played a role in reducing strokes. Every year approximately 795,000 people residing in the United States have a stroke; however, between 1996 and 2006 the rate of stroke death decreased by 33.5 percent. Thus, the total yearly deaths from stroke fell by 18.4 percent. In later years, stroke deaths also decreased. For example, in 2008 the number of stroke deaths was 133,750, while in 2007 it was 135,952. Go et al. (2014) report that stroke deaths continued to decrease from 2000 to 2010. While relative stroke deaths were decreased by 35.8 percent, there was a decline in the actual number of deaths from stroke. Despite the decline in the stroke deaths, people continue to suffer from either a new type of stroke or a recurrent one. These types are either an ischemic or hemorrhagic stroke. Studies show that approximately 15 million people all over the world suffer a stroke on a yearly basis. Of this amount, five million people are permanently disabled from the stroke (O'Shea & Goode, 2013). O'Shea and Goode (2013) further stated that in the northern part of Ireland 4,000 people are afflicted with stroke in a year. It is predicted that 700,000 people in the United States will have a stroke in one year and of the 700,000, more than 150,000 will be fatal (Alkadry et al., 2011). The leading cause of death and disability in people globally is ischemic stroke (von Sarnowski et al., 2013).

According to Zhou et al. (2014), the leading cause of death and adult disability in China is stroke. They also stated that the most lethal types of stroke are intracerebral hemorrhage (ICH), and this type is more frequently seen in Chinese populations than in western populations. In the United States stroke is the leading cause of long-term disability. In addition, 795,000 people in the United States experience the first stroke or a recurrent one every year (O'Brien et al., 2013).

Avoidable Deaths Statistics from Stroke, Hypertension, and Heart Disease in the United States

The Morbidity and Mortality Weekly Report (MMWR, 2013) documented the avoidable death statistics in U.S. people less than 75 years old with underlying conditions such as ischemic heart disease, stroke, hypertension or chronic rheumatic heart disease. The report pointed to the deaths that could be avoided from heart disease, stroke, and hypertension from 2001 to 2010. It showed that in 2010, 200,070 deaths were avoidable and the death rate was 60.7 per 100,000 people. However, in this same year, people in the older age group who were between 65 and 74 years had the highest death rates. It is important to note that 56 percent of deaths were of people less than 65 years of age. Deaths deemed avoidable were higher for males compared to females, and higher for black males in comparison to other races. Death rates were higher in black people and American Indians and Alaska Natives relative to white people, but in Hispanics, Asians and Pacific Islanders the mortality rate was lower than in whites. Nevertheless, there was a 29 percent decrease in avoidable deaths from 2001 to 2010, not only from stroke but also from heart disease and hypertensive disease.

The MMWR (2013) further reported that avoidable deaths from the aforementioned conditions varied by age, race, ethnicity, gender, place and time. Alarmingly, black death rates were almost double those of whites. Deaths that could be avoided were abundant in counties in the south census region. Also, avoidable deaths from these diseases in 2010 "ranged from 36.3 to 99.6 per 100,000 population in Minnesota and the District of Columbia," respectively, a greater than twofold difference.

Strategies to Avoid Stroke Deaths

The MMRW (2013) reports that several diseases and stroke deaths could be avoided by implementing some key strategies, such as improvement in lifestyle behaviors, treatment of risk factors, and focusing on the social determinants that contribute to health.

In the United States, 5 percent of annual deaths are from stroke. Individual lifestyle behaviors characterized as "not healthy" play a role. Lifestyle behaviors such as the use of tobacco, not enough exercise, and the consumption of a lot of alcohol are contributing factors, compounded with blood pressure that is not controlled, raised cholesterol levels, and obesity.

The MMWR (2013) stressed the importance of public health initiatives and interventions. The initiatives should be national, state and local. These initiatives should aim at efforts to address broader state issues that contribute to diseases that affect the health of people in the population. Improving health care systems and educating people to practice healthy behavioral choices to decrease avoidable deaths from heart disease, stroke and hypertension disease are some initiatives that could be considered. The initiatives would help to improve and create both healthier people and a healthier environment, thus decreasing avoidable deaths.

Mortality: Stroke

In other countries, deaths due to stroke are also a major health concern. For example, in China, 21.6 percent of the total deaths in men and 20.8 percent in women are attributed to stroke. Stroke deaths continue to be a major health concern in rural and urban areas in China (Feng et al., 2013). In Canada, stroke is reported to be the third leading cause of death. More women die from stroke than men on a yearly basis. Also, almost 315,000 people in Canada are living with conditions due to stroke (Heart and Stroke Foundation of Canada, 2014a). It is projected that stroke incidence will rise over the next twenty years (Zhong et al., 2014). However, in the United States, stroke has decreased in ranking. It used to be the third cause of death, but it is now the fourth cause of death behind other illnesses such as heart disease, cancer and chronic lower respiratory disease (Mitka, 2011).

Lifestyle Changes for Decreasing Stroke Risk

McDonnell et al. (2013) stated that adult people who implement healthy lifestyle choices can lower their risk of stroke by 80 percent in comparison to those who do not make these choices. They recommend regular physical activity as a key part of a healthy lifestyle. Importantly, since stroke deaths in the United States have been decreasing, there is a call to institute preventive measures to continue improving the falling stroke death rates. For example, Mitka (2011) suggested people adopt healthy lifestyle choices as primary preventive measures of stroke, because this is recommended by the revised guidelines by the American Heart Association and the American Stroke Association. These guidelines stress the need for people to exercise regularly, to consume a low-fat diet high in fruit and vegetables, consume alcohol in moderation, and maintain normal body weight. In addition, the guidelines call for emergency department doctors to assist in stroke prevention. The guidelines recommend that emergency departments initiate programs and interventions for smoking cessation, screen patients who arrive in the emergency department for hypertension, identify those with atrial fibrillation (a condition of abnormal heart rhythm that can lead to stroke), and assess their need for anticoagulation therapy.

Additionally, they should refer patients with drug or alcohol abuse problems to suitable therapeutic programs.

Physical Activity

The McDonnell et al. (2013) Reasons for Geographic and Racial Differences in Stroke (REGARDS) study was a national, population-based, longitudinal study that investigated whether self-reported physical activity was associated with risk of incident stroke in black and white subjects. The researchers recruited an oversample of blacks and residents of the southeastern "stroke belt," an area with the highest stroke mortality rates relative to the rest of the United States. Subjects were over 45 years of age. They were followed up every 6 months for stroke events. The researchers conducted the study from 2003 to 2007 on 30,239 subjects; 42 percent were black. They analyzed their findings on 27,348 subjects who had self-reported their frequency of moderate to vigorous physical activity at baseline. Following up with subjects for an average of 5.7 years, the researchers found 918 validated incident stroke and transient ischemic attack (TIA) cases.

"There was no significant association between PA frequency and risk of stroke by sex groups, although there was a trend toward increased risk for men reporting PA 0 to 3× a week compared with ≥ 4× a week" (McDonnell et al., 2013, p. 2519).

McDonnell et al. (2013) found no association between physical activity frequency and incident stroke/transient ischemic attack in women. They reported that there were no protective effects of physical activity on incident stroke/TIA in women who reported they had performed physical activity one to three times per week or more than four times a week. They stated that the limitations of their physical activity measure may be a possible cause for not finding an association between physical activity and incident stroke in women, because their physical activity measure did not capture walking and other low-intensity physical activity.

However, a significant difference in stroke risks was noted between the subjects who had reported physical activity one to three times or more than four times a week. This frequency of physical activity led the authors to confirm that physical activity performed regularly at moderate to heavy intensity protects against stroke and TIA.

It is the researchers' belief that physical activity has a positive effect on stroke risk factors such as diabetes, hypertension, body mass index, alcohol use and smoking. This may be due to their findings that subjects in both physical activity groups were least likely to smoke, did not have hypertension or high body mass index, and had a lower incidence of diabetes compared to those who did not exercise. This led McDonnell et al. (2013) to speculate that the decrease in stroke risk in exercising subjects may be explained partly by the positive outcomes of physical activity on conditions such as hypertension, diabetes mellitus and body mass index. They concluded that "moderate to heavy intensity physical activity is protective against stroke and TIA" (p. 2522).

Stroke Types

There are different types of strokes and their causes may be either similar or different. The Heart and Stroke Foundation of Canada (2014a) listed the two main types of stroke that are caused from blood clots and bleeding. It also lists their subtypes. The two main types of stroke are hemorrhagic and ischemic strokes. The majority of strokes are ischemic, caused by a blood clot in the brain; as a result, blood flow to the brain is interrupted. The two types of ischemic stroke are thrombotic stroke and embolic stroke. Transient Ischemic Attack (TIA), otherwise called "mini stroke," is due to a temporary interruption of blood flow to the brain.

According to Woo et al. (2013), every year in the United States, 40 to 50 percent of hemorrhagic stroke patients die within 30 days. The Heart and Stroke Foundation of Canada (2014) reports that hemorrhagic stroke results from ruptured blood vessels (bleeding not controlled) in the brain. The two main types of hemorrhagic stroke are subarachnoid hemorrhage and intracerebral hemorrhage. Importantly, these types of hemorrhagic strokes can result from blood pressure that is not controlled, as well as structural problems in the individual blood vessels in the brain.

Falcone et al. (2012) documented that of all the forms of stroke, intracerebral hemorrhage (ICH) is most severe, and it is the cause of 15 percent of acute strokes in the United States. Furthermore, hypertension is reported to be a potent risk factor for this type of stroke. Additionally, "hypertension has been associated with increased ICH volumes and worse clinical outcome" (Falcone et al., 2012, p. 2878).

It is important to know the signs of a stroke and seek prompt medical attention. The Heart and Stroke Foundation (2014) reports five signs of stroke.

- Weakness
- Difficulty speaking
- Vision problems
- Headache
- Dizziness

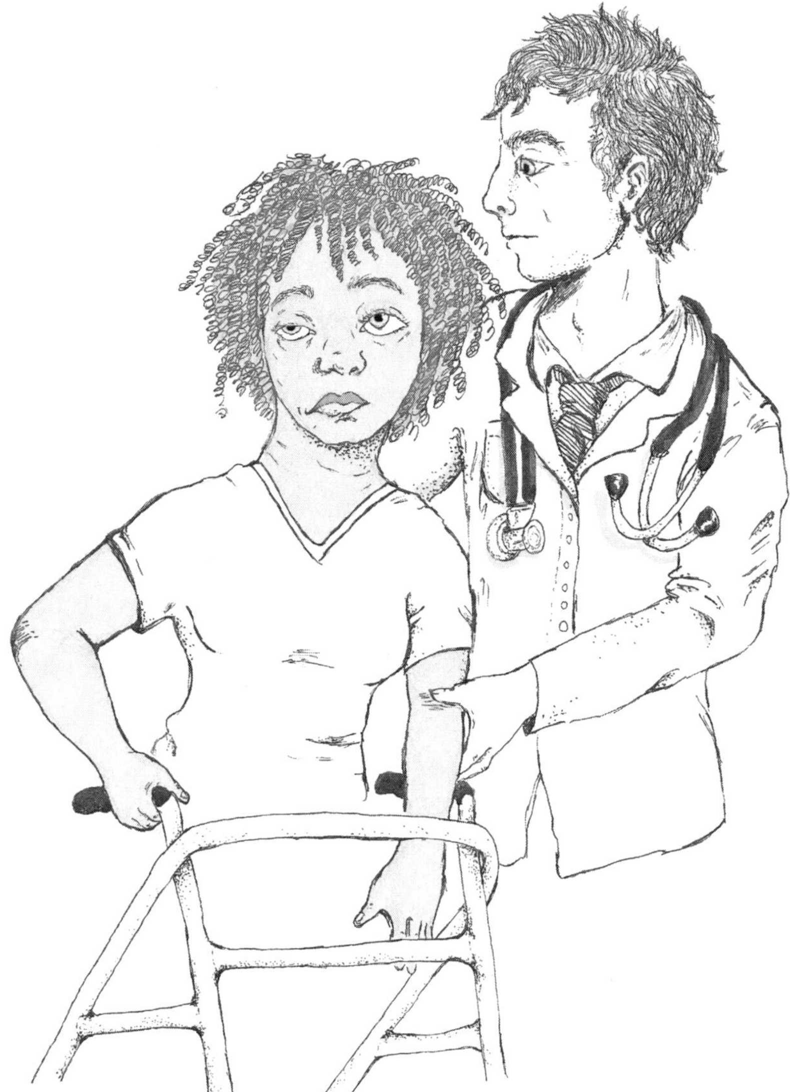

Figure 8. A person with decreased mobility after a stroke. The patient, on the left, is assisted with ambulation by a physiotherapist, on the right, to increase her mobility, balance and strength after a stroke. A low walker is used for ambulation (courtesy Dominique Diedrick).

Although some or all of these signs may be due to other health problems, they should not be ignored. According to the Heart and Stroke Foundation (2014), these stroke signs are sudden.

Figure 8 shows a person who suffered a stroke.

Economic Impact of Stroke

The impact of stroke on the individual can be devastating, and the cost to the health care system can be enormous. This is due to the varying disabilities people experience from the effects of a stroke. For example, an estimated 32,000 people live with disabilities in Northern Ireland. The disabilities are due to the effects of stroke. According to O'Shea and Goode (2013), the approximate cost to the UK economy is 8.9 billion per year as a result of stroke. While direct care accounts for 50 percent of this cost, 27 percent is for informal care.

O'Brien et al. (2013) stated that in the United States, Medicare beneficiaries (primarily people age 65 and older) account for most stroke events. They reported that even though some people may suffer a stroke and not have disabilities from the stroke, almost 40 percent of an estimated 476,000 of those who suffer a stroke every year do need post-acute care.

High Blood Pressure and Ischemic Stroke

Zhong et al. (2014) assessed the association between plasma homocysteine (Hcy), blood pressure and poor discharge outcome in subjects with acute ischemic stroke. The researchers also looked at whether high homocysteine (hHcy) would increase the risk of poor outcome based on subjects' high blood pressure status.

The study was carried out from June 1, 2009, to May 31, 2013, in three hospitals in northern cites in China. Subjects had a clinical diagnosis of acute ischemic stroke. The study consisted of 3,695 subjects in total. Of this number, 2,381 were males and 1,314 were females. Their average age was 62.4 years. Subjects were divided into four subgroups based on their blood pressure levels and their concentration of Hcy. The groups were (1) nonhigh blood pressure with nonhigh Hcy (nhHcy), (2) nonhigh blood pressure with hHcy, (3) high blood pressure with nhHcy, and (4) high blood pressure with hHcy.

The authors found that high plasma Hcy concentration was an independent risk factor for prognosis in subjects with acute ischemic stroke. Blood pressure was also found to be an independent risk factor, and hHcy may have helped to increase the risk of poor outcome in subjects with high blood pressure. The author elaborated that their findings are consistent with a study done by Pniewski, Chodakowska-Zebrowska, Wozniak, Stepien and Stafiej (2003), which investigated how Hcy level influenced the prognosis of stroke at the start of a stroke. Additionally, Pniewski et al. (2003) found that mild hyperhomocysteinemia (over 15 umol\L) may have increased the risk of poor recovery in stroke patients.

Zhong et al. (2014) indicate that homocysteine may raise blood pressure levels; as a result, arterial stiffness may occur. The arterial stiffness may be related to decreased vascular endothelial integrity and decreasing efficiency of vasodilation.

Hypertension is also a risk factor of stroke in other ethnic groups. For example, Tang et al. (2014) conducted a study in Inner Mongolia, an autonomous region in north China. This study was carried out from June 2003 to July 2012 on subjects 20 years old and older. The purpose "was to evaluate the effect of hypertension and alcohol drinking on stroke incidence." They also looked at whether drinking alcohol would increase the risk of stroke in those subjects who had hypertension. In the follow-up period, the researchers looked at stroke incidence among study groups. Of 120 subjects, 76 ischemic stroke subjects and 44 hemorrhagic stroke subjects were examined. This study used four subgroups: (1) nonhypertension/nondrinkers, (2) nonhypertension/drinkers, (3) hypertension/drinkers, and (4) hypertension/nondrinkers.

The result of the study showed "that hypertension was the most prevalent risk factor for stroke" (p. 3), and this was noted in greater than a third of subjects. For instance, hypertension/nondrinkers' and hypertension/drinkers' risk for stroke was significantly higher when compared to other subgroups such as nonhypertension/nondrinkers. Similarly, individuals who had hypertension and were drinkers were more likely to have a stroke. During the follow-up period, which was 10 years, the cumulative incidence rate of stroke was 1.5, 2.8, 7.4 and 12.5 percent. This was observed in subjects in all subgroups. Notably, subjects who had hypertension and were either in the drinking group or nondrinking group were likely to be elderly. Not only were they elders, but their histories included several illnesses. For example, their family histories of cardiovascular disease and total cholesterol were higher. Those who had hypertension and were drinkers were most likely to be men.

The researcher pointed to similar studies. Higashiyama et al. (2013) found that in Japanese men, both total stroke and ischemic stroke risk were the highest among drinkers. Tang et al. (2014) reported on the British Regional Heart 20-year follow-up study by Emberson et al. (2005), which showed that subjects who were heavy drinkers had a 74 percent higher risk of a major coronary event, as well as a 133 percent higher risk of stroke, than subjects who were occasional drinkers.

Tang et al. (2014) concluded that there is a need for further prospective study. The study should include a larger sample size to observe the cumulative effective of drinking and hypertension, and its effects on the incidence of stroke.

Genetic Variation and Intracerebral Hemorrhage

Falcone et al. (2012) researched individuals of European ancestry in a prospective multicenter case-control study. Of 2,275 participants, 1,025 were patients and 1,247 were control participants. Study participants were over 18 years of age.

The purpose of the study was to investigate whether the burden of blood pressure-related single nucleotide polymorphisms was associated with risk of intracerebral hemorrhage (ICH) and pre–ICH diagnosis of hypertension. Falcone and others stated that many common genetic variants or single nucleotide polymorphisms have been linked to blood pressure levels. Thus, the authors believed that genetic risk scores (GRSs) would provide an aggregated measure of the burden of risk alleles due to high blood pressure carried by each person.

The study revealed that the burden of risk alleles for blood pressure was linked with risk of ICH. It is important to note that risk of alleles was measured by the GRSs, which were found to be associated with clinically identified pre–ICH hypertension. The relationship between GRS and ICH risk seemed to be formed by ICH in deep regions of the brain. There was a stronger association among participants who were not considered hypertensive.

Their study is the first to show that genetic variants for blood pressure also drive risk of ICH. Also, their study supports previous studies that show the viability of applying GRSs to stroke. It is their belief that there is not a single nucleotide polymorphism variant in relation to hypertension that is associated with ICH, but rather it is the aggregate burden of the variants at the end point that puts people at greater risk of ICH. According to the researchers, their findings are vital for risk prediction. Because there is not a lot of acute treatment for people who have an ICH, it is crucial to recognize those who are high risk for getting an ICH. If these people are identified, there is a possibility for implementing aggressive preventive strategies.

The Ethnic/Racial Variations of Intracerebral Hemorrhage (ERICH) study is a multicenter, prospective, large case-control study of ICH. ERICH was carried out by Woo et al. (2013). The purpose was to identify the genetic variation that affect risk of ICH in non–Hispanic whites, non-Hispanic blacks and Hispanics. The researchers also wanted to understand how risk factors and imaging characteristics specific to race and ethnicity were distributed.

Disparities in Stroke Risks

The prevalence of stroke is higher in some groups than others. For instance, in the United States minorities have a higher incidence and prevalence of stroke (Gutierrez & Williams, 2014). Howard, Carson, Holmes and Kaufman (2009) conducted the REGARDS study on 27,748 black and white subjects between 2003 and 2007 and followed them through 2011. Subjects were 45 years old and older. Black people were oversampled for this study, as well as people from the "southern stroke belt," from Georgia, Arkansas, Louisiana, North Carolina, and other states. The researchers wanted to address whether differential elevated systolic blood pressure levels were associated with greater stroke risk in black subjects compared to their white counterparts. This was specific to adults 45 to 65 years of age. The authors used this age group because they believed that the racial disparities in stroke risk exist more for black people in this age group than other minority race or ethnic groups.

The finding demonstrated that 71 percent of blacks were hypertensive while 51 percent of whites were hypertensive. But black subjects had the lowest odds of controlled blood pressure, even though their awareness of hypertension was greater. For black subjects, average achieved blood pressure was almost 5 mm Hg higher in comparison to white subjects.

The 4.5-year follow-up study revealed that among 27,780 subjects, 715 stroke events happened. A systolic blood pressure difference of 10 mm Hg was associated with an 8 percent increased stroke risk in white subjects, while in blacks it was 24 percent.

For all systolic blood pressure levels, the risk of stroke on a whole was two to three times more in black subjects than white subjects. Excessive stroke risk was shown in the age group 45 to 64 and was seen in those with stage 1 hypertension, which corresponds to systolic levels between 140 and 159 mm Hg. Of these, 1067 (18 percent) were black subjects and a lower percentage (10 percent) were white subjects.

Nonetheless, this study did not show any evidence "of a racial disparity in the risk of incident stroke among normotensive individuals" (p. 50) regardless of age. Additionally, stroke risk overall was higher in subjects 65 to 74 years of age, but this was not a dramatic difference.

The authors believed that their findings regarding the racial disparity in stroke risk among subjects 45 to 64 years of age could be considerably decreased, for example, by improving blood pressure control. Blood pressure control may help to decrease "the long standing racial disparity in stroke risks in the United States" (p. 51).

In order to determine whether racial and ethnic disparities in the prevalence of stroke are explained by the suboptimal control of cardiovascular risk factors in the United States, Gutierrez and Williams (2014) utilized data from the National Health and Nutrition Examination Survey. Data was gathered from 2000 to 2009 from the noninstitutionalized U.S. population. The study analyzed data for individuals who were 20 years old or older. Subjects were non–Hispanic whites (NHW), non–Hispanic blacks (NHB), and Mexican Americans (MA). This sample consisted of 37,847 subjects, of which 49 percent were male. In terms of race and ethnicity, 79 percent of subjects were NHW, 12 percent NHB, and 9 percent were MA.

The analysis showed that in comparison to NHW subjects, NHB subjects had higher physical inactivity, obesity, smoking, hypertension and diabetes mellitus. In contrast, MA subjects had a lower prevalence of hypertension, smoking, and hypercholesterolemia compared to NHW, but physical inactivity and diabetes were higher. Alarmingly, NHB and MA hypertensive subjects were more likely to report suboptimal control of their blood pressure compared to their NHW counterparts; the percentage for NHB subjects was 87 percent while it was 83 percent for NHW. Reported suboptimal hypertension control was 90 percent for MA. Although this analysis consisted of only 12 percent NHB, stroke health disparities were shown to be more prevalent and higher in most self-reported categories for NHB subjects compared to the other groups, especially NHW. For instance, NHW subjects had a higher prevalence of hypercholesterolemia, but it was often not controlled in NHB at a rate of 74 percent, compared to 69 percent for NHW and 79 percent for MA subjects. Again, although the total stroke prevalence was 2.1 percent, a greater frequency of stroke was shown among NHB subjects compared to NHW. But stroke was least common in MA subjects.

Nonetheless, other factors combined with ethnicity and racial disparities were shown. A number of suboptimal vascular risk factors were identified. For example, stroke was observed to be more frequent as subjects' age increased. Other risk factors were "physical inactivity, smoking, suboptimal hypertension control, suboptimal diabetes control, and suboptimal hypercholesterolemia control" (p. 1082).

The authors pointed to the degree of difficulty health care providers are confronted with in the United States due to various suboptimal vascular risk factors. The risk of stroke is greater in those whose blood pressure and diabetes mellitus are not controlled when compared to subjects who have these conditions controlled or do not have these existing risk factors.

These findings are very concerning. There is a grave need to decrease hypertension prevalence and institute primary preventive measures in community-based organizations in every state. The emphasis should be directed to at-risk populations. Rigorous control of risk factors, such as hypertension and diabetes mellitus, among the U.S. population would play a huge role in improving health. These measures are important and particularly relevant for blacks due to their alarming rates of hypertension and diabetes. If these risk factors are minimized, it is likely that the rising stroke prevalence and its disparity could be decreased or prevented.

Education to increase awareness is also significant. Education should be directed at a broader level. This should include hypertension control, as well as measures to prevent and decrease disability and deaths from stroke. Policy planners play a key role in addressing any existing disparities and socioeconomic variables, especially in ethnic groups. The hope is to decrease or eliminate disparities with the implementation of strategic programs and preventive interventions. It would be even more beneficial to evaluate programs yearly or every other year to look at progress and determine whether intervention modification is needed.

One key measure to decreasing stroke risk is adequate blood pressure control. But according to Hatori et al. (2014), target blood pressure is not often achieved despite hypertension management guidelines advancement and useful blood pressure medication. Their study investigated changes in clinical practices related to controlling blood pressure in hypertensive subjects according to 2009 guidelines in Kanagawa Prefecture. This research was conducted from 2008 to 2011. The researchers collected data from 675 subjects in 2008, 332 in 2009, and 1076 in 2011. Subjects were assigned to groups, and an analysis examined where office-measured blood pressure targets were and were not achieved.

The findings showed that office-measured systolic blood pressure was decreased. For instance, there was a reduction in office blood pressure from 2008 to 2011. The improvement in achieving target blood pressure was also found to be effective. For example, the target achievement rate was 23.6 percent in 2008, 36.6 percent in 2009, and 41.2 percent in 2011. Notably, nonelderly subjects younger than 65 years of age had a higher control rate of office-measured blood pressure. For example it was 41.2 percent in 2011 compared to 23.6 percent in 2008. The authors speculate that specific antihypertensive agents, such as angiotensin II receptor blockers (ARBs), which were used by more subjects in 2011, probably explain the improvement.

Their findings led them to believe that for blood pressure to be adequately controlled, blood pressure medication treatment needs to be more aggressive. Of interest, the highest prescribed antihypertensive agent was the calcium channel blocker (CCB), and it was the highest every year during the study period. Not surprisingly, Hatori et al. (2014) stated that "CCBs are the first-line antihypertensive medications in Japan" (p. 26).

Since blacks and Hispanics who live in the United States are disproportionately affected by ICH, and the onset of this condition appears to happen at a younger age compared to whites (Woo et al., 2013), there is a desperate need to examine factors that contribute to the racial differences. The annual incidence for ICH is 48.9 percent for black people, but in whites it is 26.6 percent. For Hispanic people in the United States, ICH is double that of non–Hispanic whites.

Lifestyle changes may help to decrease both ischemic stroke and TIA. Von Sarnowski, Putaala, Grittner et al. (2013) studied patients 18 to 55 years of age with cerebrovascular events. Patients were Europeans. The purpose was to determine patients' prevalence of cerebrovascular events. An analysis of patients with ischemic stroke and TIA was also performed to explain sex- and age-specific risk factors.

Of the 5023 enrolled subjects, 1071 had TIA, 3396 had ischemic stroke and 271 had ICH. This study analyzed 4467 patients with ischemic stroke or TIA, of which 59.4 percent were men. Female patients were younger than male patients. The findings showed a high frequency of well-documented cerebrovascular risk factors. The most frequent well-documented risk factors and modifiable factors were observed in men: for example, smoking, physical inactivity, arterial hypertension, dyslipidemia, alcohol consumption and short sleep duration. Smoking percentage was high for men, an alarming 55 percent. Physical inactivity (48.2 percent) and arterial hypertension (46.6 percent) were also high. The proportion of men 45 years and older with four or more well-documented and modifiable risk factors was 29.0 percent; for women, it was 20.3 percent. Men were found to be more overweight compared to women, even though a prevalence of obesity was shown in both. However, abdominal obesity was frequently observed in women, and it was reported to be excessive in almost three-fourths of those age 25 years and older. Women were also physically less active than men. This physical inactivity was documented in women 35 years old or younger, but women less than 25 years old were also less active.

The findings also showed modifiable less well-documented or potentially modifiable risk factors. For instance, high risk of alcohol intake and migraine were most frequently seen in men. But in comparison to women the only significant prevalent risk factor was migraine (26.5 percent), noted in those 25 years and older. Because of the study outcome, the authors emphasized the importance to increase awareness of modifiable risk factors with a focus on younger populations with stroke.

Eames, Hoffmann, and Phillips (2014) examined 77 stroke subjects' recall and recognition of risk factors; subjects reported performance and stage of change for stroke risk-related behaviors within 3 months after they were discharged from hospital. The authors utilized a brief educational intervention model to carry out their study. This model was patient centered with educational information tailored to the needs of each subject. The study was carried out in Australia. Subjects were assigned to either the intervention group (40) or the control group (37).

The researchers found that there was no significant difference between both groups for the outcomes measured. Subjects increased recall of personal and general risk factors; however, low awareness of risk factors was still present. For example, the majority of subjects had recalled between one and three risk factors during the follow-up period. Interestingly, subjects' recognition of risk factors was reduced during the baseline of the study and follow–up period.

The findings also revealed a progression from a nonaction to action category. This was noted in five of the seven behaviors, such as "healthy eating, maintaining a healthy weight, taking medication, and having regular medical checks" (p. 560).

Despite the improvement, the change was not significant between baselines and follow-up, for instance, in behaviors such as subjects carrying out regular physical activity, reducing smoking and reducing the consumption of alcohol. It is the authors' belief that their 3-month intervention study did not provide extra benefits to subjects outside the usual care.

Effects After Stroke

Few studies have followed patients for greater than two to three years after a stroke. Brunborg and Ytrehus (2013) conducted a qualitative interview study on nine patients who had survived a stroke. Participants provided descriptive factors about their adaptation and subjective well-being 10 years after their stroke. The age of participants was between 60 and 90 years old.

The researchers found that despite participants' decreased functional levels, a majority of them had adapted well and had a positive attitude by accepting the changes in their life following the stroke. Most participants stated that a positive adaptation to their situation following the stroke was made possible based on their personal attitudes and characteristics. For example, their strong will power and positive attitudes played a role in their adaptation after the stroke.

In terms of activities, many participants were unable to carry out tasks they used to perform before they experienced the stroke. However, they tried to adapt by seeking other new activities that they found meaningful. For example, many participants had hobbies that allowed them to concentrate on positive activities and interact with others.

Those who suffered cognitive impairments had adapted to their decreased memory and difficulty with speaking. For example, they adapted by writing down messages and appointments.

Many participants used social networks as a way to engage in activities that were meaningful. Although social networks and family were viewed as positive factors, participants' characteristics were vital to how they adapted. Nevertheless, a majority of participants had stated that their spouses, family and friends were the most important factors that contributed to their well-being.

Financial impact was a challenge for some participants. One participant had to retire early due to the stroke but saw this as a requirement for changing habits. For example, the extra time the participant had after retiring fully resulted in a positive change. Additionally, two participants found it difficult financially after stroke. The financial strain poses great difficulty for the youngest participant, who had suffered a stroke when he was 48 years old. This participant had expressed concerns about his 12-year-old dependent, and he continued to experience financial difficulty 10 years after stroke.

Several participants found stroke to result in a positive change, providing new opportunities, especially in their dietary habits. They engaged in healthier lifestyle changes after the stroke than they did prior to the stroke. It was reported that many participants had obtained knowledge on how to prevent a new stroke and prevent adverse health conditions and disease. They viewed the stroke "as a wakeup call" (p. 1058), and they had concerns about lifestyle preventive activities such as physical activity level, diet, and alcohol and cigarette use. Eight participants expressed concerns about a healthy diet. Participants who had smoked before their stroke had quit smoking.

Public assistance was important for many participants. They received this type of support when they were first discharged from hospital following the stroke. But one participant lacked energy and motivation to start training independently. At the time of the study few participants had stroke-related support.

This study suggests the need for continued financial and social support for stroke victims, many years after stroke. Policy planners play an important role in providing programs, interventions and available community resources to assist these individuals. These measures will probably help to increase stroke survivors' adaptation levels and behaviors to cope and manage with the consequences of stroke emotionally, physically and financially. Strategies should not only focus on younger people after stroke, but older people should be included, because they may be more vulnerable. "As older people are often left with some form of permanent disability, many studies have focused on functional recovery and physical rehabilitation" (Jayasekara, 2009, p. 966).

In a similar study, Lakshminarayan et al. (2014) examined the trends in stroke survival in the early period after stroke and over the long term. Trends were examined by stroke subtype, such as ischemic or hemorrhagic strokes. The researcher reported the 10-year post-stroke survival outcomes that pertained to the 1995 and 2000 surveys and contrasted them to 1980s and 1990s post-stroke survival. This Minnesota Stroke Survey utilized all patients who were hospitalized with an acute stroke. Their ages ranged from 30 to 74 years of age.

There were 3773 reported acute stroke events, 55 percent to 70 percent of which were confirmed as such by the World Health Organization (WHO) definition of stroke. Neuroimaging showed that 75 to 81 percent were ischemic strokes. There was an improved ten-year long-term ischemic stroke survival, and this was observed from 1990 to 2000 for both men and women. For example, in men, survival was 35.3 percent in 1990 and 50 percent in 2000; in women, it was 38 percent in 1990, and 55.3 percent in 2000.

In terms of hemorrhagic stroke survival, improvement was observed in both men and women, but the trends in hemorrhagic stroke improvement were not significant. The researchers believed that the small numbers of hemorrhagic stroke may be a factor in the improved trends results. The findings also revealed improvement in early and long-term age-adjusted post-stroke survival in men and women between 1980 and 2000. It was noted that survival had improved in those with severe strokes. This was especially seen in individuals who were admitted to hospital with major deficits. Individuals admitted to hospitals unconscious and with neurological deficits had decreased from 1980 to 2000.

The researchers believed that the post-stroke survival trends may be due to several factors, such as detection of less severe events or improved care in early survival. Additionally, "the observed improvement in long-term survival is likely a reflection of increased use of secondary preventive therapies and especially improved hypertension awareness and treatment" (p. 2580), as well as improvement in the overall health of the population and people living longer.

Life satisfaction after a stroke is important for stroke survivors. Boosman, Schepers, Post and Viesser-Meily (2011) examined life satisfaction for three groups of participants. These were socially inactive, moderately active and highly active participants. The authors further examined the extent to which social activity was associated with their satisfaction 3 years after a stroke. The participants were admitted to four rehabilitation centers in the Netherlands. The researchers analyzed their study findings on a total of 165 participants. Of this number, two participants had resided in a nursing home and 163 had lived alone.

The researchers found that participants who were less socially active were older, commonly lived with a partner, and received less social support, and their cognition and daily living functioning (ADL) were worse. Nearly 68 percent (112 participants) were satisfied with their life as a whole.

In terms of life satisfaction between the three groups, the socially inactive group was found to be less satisfied with life as a whole, including sexual life and their ability for self-care.

Interestingly, it was revealed that life satisfaction was due to both social activity and ADL functioning, but it was least related to social support and cognitive functioning. Additionally, social activity was "a significant predictor of life satisfaction" (p. 465) 3 years post-stroke. Nevertheless, limited social activities have been linked with declining life satisfaction. Importantly, the findings showed that sexual life and financial and vocational situations had the lowest satisfaction rate, but satisfaction rate was higher for family life and partner relationship.

The researchers noted that their study was carried out in a rehabilitation setting. They stated that "patients selected for rehabilitation are relatively young" (p. 466); because of the younger age of the patients, they may have had more involvement in social activities, leading to higher life satisfaction. They stressed the importance of patients remaining involved in social activities, even after their rehabilitation phase.

Part II

7

Nonpharmacological Management for Hypertension

People with hypertension can modify their lifestyles for effective blood pressure control by changing their dietary and physical behaviors and taking their blood pressure medication as prescribed.

People diagnosed with hypertension need to take prescribed medications to treat and control their blood pressure and prevent hypertension-related complications. But it is well documented that for some people with hypertension, blood pressure is not adequately controlled. Disproportionate rates of uncontrolled blood pressure and its clinical results have been reported for African Americans compared to whites (Ameling et al., 2014; Warren-Findlow et al., 2012). The literature frequently describes many reasons for uncontrolled blood pressure in the population. The associated organ damage related to poorly controlled blood pressure is also widely documented. Ma et al. (2011) stated that low treatment adherence is the main cause for uncontrolled blood pressure, which is an estimated 29 to 59 percent in clinical practice.

Despite pharmacological management of hypertension many people still have uncontrolled blood pressure. Lack of adherence to dietary restrictions and medication regimes are two impediments to hypertension control (Gross et al., 2013). As such, two key ways people can modify their lifestyle behaviors for effective blood pressure control are by changing their dietary and physical behaviors and by taking their blood pressure medication as prescribed. People should not perceive lifestyle changes as temporary; they need to continuously adhere to an antihypertensive long-term lifestyle regime, because hypertension is a chronic disease.

Nonpharmacological hypertension management, for instance dietary changes and exercise programs, can also enhance the effectiveness of blood pressure medication and improve overall health. Given the magnitude of illnesses caused in part from uncontrolled hypertension, it is crucial that people with this chronic condition take special interest in their health. As a result, risks of hypertensive-related illnesses could be prevented or decreased. Global deaths, especially from cardiovascular disease, could also be minimized. If people make an effort to implement behavioral interventions, the positive results would likely be better blood pressure control, decreased hypertension-related illnesses, and a healthier and longer lifespan.

Behavioral lifestyle interventions (for example, weight reduction, improved dietary measures, increased exercise and management of stress and anger) are reported to have an overall beneficial result on blood pressure (Ma et al., 2011).

This chapter will focus on nonpharmacological measures for hypertension management. It will highlight research findings that focus on lifestyle modifications for blood pressure control and management.

Individual Lifestyle Modifications for Hypertension Management

Why Decrease Sodium and Increase Intake of Fruits and Vegetables?

A genetic sensitivity to salt, which is high in certain populations, is a significant risk factor for hypertension. In addition, a high-sodium diet has been reported to be a major risk factor for hypertension (Gu et al., 2013) even in people resistant to salt. Nonadherence to medication is also one of the reported causes for uncontrolled blood pressure (Leung et al., 2012). Lifestyle interventions that can have an effect on controllable risk factors for hypertension are: lose weight (if overweight), consume more fruit and vegetables, decrease intake of sodium, exercise more, and drink alcohol in moderation (Kolasa, Solid, Smith Edge, & Bouchoux, 2012). It is important for people to consume a variety of fruit and vegetables daily. This is to ensure they are getting sufficient nutrients to meet their daily requirements. Figure 9 shows a variety of fruits people can include in their daily diets.

According to Fernandez et al. (2011), lifestyle interventions such as decreased consumption of salt; increased consumption of fruits, fiber, vegetables, low-fat dairy; decreased intake of saturated and total fat; more physical activity; and weight reduction have been shown to significantly reduce blood pressure. Folson, Parker and Harnack (2007) stated that the National High Blood Pressure Education Program and the American Heart Association widely recommended the Dietary Approaches to Stop Hypertension (DASH) diet to decrease blood pressure. The DASH diet focuses on decreased intake of sodium, increased intake of fruits and vegetables, and consumption of dairy products that are low in fat. "It includes whole grains, poultry, fish, and nuts and is reduced in fats, red meat, sweets, and sugar-containing beverages" (Folson et al., 2007, p. 225). It is also high in fiber (Woolf & Bisognano, 2011).

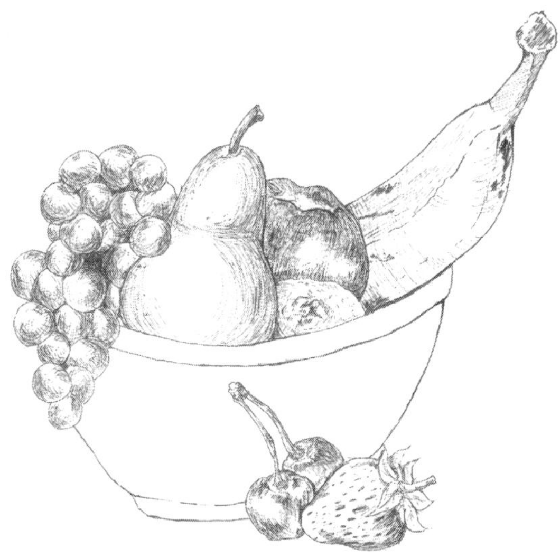

Figure 9. Fruits are healthy food choices and should be part of everyone's daily intake (courtesy Dominique Diedrick).

Because increased sodium intake is a risk factor for hypertension, it would benefit people to limit their daily sodium intake. There are some people who are more sensitive to salt than others due to genetic factors. For instance, studies show that several genetic variants are linked to salt sensitivity, and this has been observed in people of different ethnicities (Gu et al., 2013). As such, it is suggested that efforts to decrease sodium consumption globally should be complemented by targeting people who are more sensitive to sodium (Gu et al., 2013).

Nevertheless, people with hypertension should refrain from adding salt to their diet. The decrease in the consumption of salt combined with the adoption of the DASH diet is likely to further decrease individuals' blood pressure (Woolf & Bisognano, 2011).

Blacks should be more careful in consuming salt or adding extra salt to their diets because of their higher rates of hypertension. "Older age, female sex, elevated baseline blood pressure, and family history of hypertension have been associated with salt sensitivity" (Gu et al., 2013, p. 501).

Kolasa et al. (2012) stated that the 2010 Dietary Guidelines for Americans (DGA) suggested a decrease in sodium to less than 2300 milligrams (mg) daily for some people and for persons 51 years or older. The authors further suggested that for any age group of African Americans, and for those with conditions like hypertension, diabetes, or chronic kidney disease, the sodium intake should be less than 1500 mg per day. Kolasa et al. (2012) note that the DGA recommendations regarding sodium intake for the population have changed. In 2005, the DGA recommended a sodium intake restriction of 2300 mg per day. But awareness and concern regarding sodium, new scientific studies, and willingness by food manufacturers and food service providers to decrease sodium have all played a role in the increased attention to sodium in public policy and the media. This led to the DGA 2010 sodium restriction of 1500 mg per day in 70 percent of the population (Kolasa et al., 2012).

It is important to note that in 2009 and 2011, the International Food Information Council (IFIC) conducted consumer research to assess awareness and behavior about sodium and blood pressure. The IFIC also gathered roundtable experts in the fall of 2010, consisting of leaders in the fields of health and nutrition. The purpose was to look at the most useful ways "to prevent or manage high blood pressure through positive lifestyle strategies" (Kolasa et al., 2012, p. 184).

The Roundtable Recommendation for Blood Pressure Management: The Lifestyle Approach

According to Kolasa et al. (2012), the roundtable discussed other lifestyle methods for blood pressure management instead of decreasing sodium alone. They pointed to the efforts of restaurants and industries that package food to decrease sodium in food, and the difficulty for consumers to follow a sodium restriction of 1500 mg per day. They believe people are more likely to achieve their blood pressure goal with multiple strategies, rather than only decreasing sodium. As such, the roundtable experts recommended a comprehensive lifestyle approach for blood pressure management, a message important for both consumers and health professionals.

The roundtable experts focused their discussion on people who are hypertensive and those at risk for the disease, and they believed that messages and strategies should be developed to target various consumer groups. Kolasa et al. (2012) reported that the roundtable experts suggested effective yet underutilized strategies to manage blood pressure. These strategies are "managing weight, consuming more fruits and vegetables, being physically active, and moderating alcohol intake" (p. 184), but the highest priorities are the first three strategies.

Nevertheless, it is still vital that people practice reading the table of nutritional facts on all food labels. People should pay special attention to the sodium (salt) value. Systolic blood pressure decreased by an average of 5.5 mm Hg with the DASH diet. Additionally, in patients with hypertension, their systolic blood pressure reduction average was 11.4 mm Hg (Woolf & Bisognano, 2011). Since multiple factors play a role in blood pressure management, a combination of lifestyle interventions would more likely benefit people with high blood pressure than create harm. The potential benefit would be adequate blood pressure control.

Salt intake and its effect on people with hypertension have been documented in other studies. Perin, Cornelio, Rodrigues and Gallani (2013) evaluated the relationship between salt consumption and sociodemographic and clinical characteristics among 108 participants with hypertension according to the following behaviors.

1. Addition of a maximum of 4 grams of salt in the preparing of meals
2. Avoiding adding salt to foods that have been prepared (avoiding using salt at the table)
3. Avoiding the consumption of foods, particularly processed foods, with a high content of salt

Participants self-reported their behaviors about salt consumption.

For clarification purposes, sociodemographic and clinical characteristics about participants were gathered, including "age, sex, color, schooling, martial situation, employment situation, individual and family income, length of time of the hypertension diagnosis" (Perin et al., 2013, p. 1015), and others.

Perin et al. (2013) found that for behavior two, most participants did not add salt to food that was already prepared, nor did they add salt at the table. The measured sodium consumption for behaviors one and three that identified the urinary sodium excretion of 209.3 mEq/24h indicated a mean consumption of daily salt of 12.1 grams.

Discretionary salt was reported to be the main source of salt consumption, representing almost 62 percent of all the salt consumed. Participants with higher sodium excretion had a lower monthly income compared to those with low excretion of sodium, and their BMI was found to be higher. BMI was an important clinical variable because it showed a connection with almost all the measurements of salt consumption, such as urinary sodium, self-reported salt intake, and total salt intake; the higher the participant's BMI, the higher their salt consumption.

For behavior one, it was shown that as women's level of schooling increased, women who cooked added less salt when they prepared foods. However, it was more common for men to have higher levels of salt consumption compared to women participants.

White participants often consumed foods with a high salt content more than participants who were not white. Participants who were considered professionally inactive had a greater salt intake compared to professional participants who were active or those who were homemakers. In addition, higher urinary sodium was positively correlated with greater ventricular mass, and higher reported intake of food with high sodium content was associated with higher participant diastolic blood pressure. Interestingly, in terms of behavior one and "number of medications and systolic blood pressure" (p. 1020), it was shown that the greater the number of medications used by female participants, and the higher their systolic blood pressure, the more they limit salt when preparing foods.

The findings show that education regarding salt consumption is needed to increase awareness and knowledge of the effects of consuming too much salt and the impact on blood pressure levels and BMI levels. Since "obesity is associated with more severe and treatment-resistant hypertension, which may be due, in part, to the increased activation of the renin-angiotensin system" (Ofili, Zappe, Purkayastha, Samuel, & Sowers, 2013, p. 3), weight reduction could probably help people keep their blood pressure controlled.

An Overview of the GenSalt Study

Gu et al. (2013) conducted the GenSalt study on Chinese adults; they looked at how blood pressure responded to dietary sodium and potassium interventions as continuous traits at both initial and follow-up studies 4.4 years apart.

For both the initial and follow-up study, the researchers utilized the dietary sodium and potassium intervention. This intervention protocol included a 7-day low-sodium feeding, a 7-day high-sodium feeding, and a 7-day high-sodium feeding with oral potassium supplementation.

After 3 days of baseline observation, subjects were given a low-salt diet (3 grams of salt or 51.3 mmol of sodium daily) for a week, followed by a high-salt diet (18 grams of salt or 307.8 mmol of sodium per day) for 7 days. Urine specimens were obtained on three occasions at baseline and at each phase of the intervention: one at 24 hours and two overnight. A 24-hr urine analysis for sodium potassium and creatinine (to ensure it was a 24-hr sample) were performed to check whether study subjects were in compliance with the dietary sodium and potassium intake. Subjects were instructed not to consume any foods that were not part of the study. Urinary output of sodium and potassium collected overnight were converted to 24-hour values using the GenSalt study formulas. High-salt diets were maintained by subjects in the final week of the study, and they also had a 60-mmol potassium (potassium chloride) supplement each day. In the study population, dietary sodium intake average was approximately 240 mmol daily.

Subjects' blood pressure was taken every morning of the 3-day baseline examination, and on the fifth, sixth, and seventh day of each intervention time frame. It is important to note that the same blood pressure equipment was used at the same time every day for each subject during the entire study period. They were instructed to "avoid alcohol, cigarette smoking, coffee/tea, and to exercise for more than 30 minutes before" having their blood pressure measured.

The study showed that blood pressure responses to dietary sodium and potassium interventions in both the initial and repeated study carried out 4.4 years later were highly correlated and significant. For instance, the correlation coefficients for systolic blood pressure levels at baseline were 0.73 to 0.80, from 0.75 to 0.82 during low-sodium interventions, 0.77 to 0.83 during high sodium, and 0.79 to 0.85 during high sodium and the supplementation of potassium intervention. Subjects' 24-hour urinary sodium and potassium output at baseline and while dietary interventions were performed showed excellent dietary sodium and potassium interventions in both studies.

The findings according to Gu et al. (2013) showed that blood pressure responses to dietary sodium and potassium interventions have long-term reproducibility and stable characteristics and potential importance for clinical and public health implications.

Adherence Interventions: Lifestyle Modifications, Medicine and Home Blood Pressure Monitoring

Uzun et al. (2009) stated that studies related to adherence or compliance to hypertension treatments often direct attention to only pharmacological interventions. They believed that reasons for nonadherence to one intervention may be different from another intervention. Therefore, the interventions should be individually assessed.

Uzun et al. (2009) examined 150 participants in Turkey. They were at least 20 years of age and had hypertension. Ninety-four of the 150 were women. The participants were on a follow-up list of outpatient clinics in the cardiology department for at least one year. Uzun et al. (2009) assessed participants for adherence to medicine, lifestyle modifications, and home blood pressure monitoring. Five categories were used to assess participants' adherence, and the definitions for each category are as follows:

1. Medicine-related adherence
2. Diet-related adherence
3. Exercise-related adherence

4. Measurement-related adherence
5. Smoking–related adherence

The study found that adherence rate was low in participants. In term of medicine-related adherence, medicine-related nonadherence was found in 28 percent of participants. Diet-related adherence was better in participants with higher education, those who were informed about their medicine, and those who were exercising. However, nonadherence to diet was 35 percent.

Exercise-related adherence was found to be better in participants with higher levels of education and those who adhered to their diet and medicine. Alarmingly, the measurement-related adherence was also found to be related to participants' education levels and how informed they were about medicine. Of interest, home blood pressure values, instead of clinic-measured blood pressure values, were predictive of target organ damage, but a significant number of participants had not taken their blood pressure at home even though they were encouraged to do so. The authors believe that cognitive differences in participants with lower levels of education may be the reason for inadequacy of adherence in these individuals.

The study also revealed that smoking-related adherence was related to age and education. In terms of age, older was better, and regarding education, lower was better. Furthermore, the disparity in income of participants was alarming. It was found to be low in 18 percent, 73 percent intermediate, and high in only 9 percent. Twenty-nine percent of participants smoked, and combined smoking and drinking was reported in only 5 percent. Apart from hypertension, participants also had diabetes mellitus, coronary artery disease, cerebrovascular accident, osteoarthritis, depression, and chronic obstructive lung disease.

The study suggests that participants' socioeconomic status and their lower education levels may have played a role in adherence to medicine and lifestyle modifications. For example, Schoenthaler et al. (2009) studied medication adherence in an underserved low-income African American population. Income may have been a factor in why subjects were unable to purchase certain foods, thus negatively affecting their adherence level.

People would benefit from education to increase their knowledge and awareness about hypertension. Education regarding the importance of taking medication and the consumption of a variety of nutritious foods from different food groups for hypertension control should be emphasized. Education should not only be directed toward people with hypertension, but those at risk for developing hypertension. Most of all, community agencies and policy planners should consider people at all levels of socioeconomic development and implement policies to minimize disparities.

Intervention Approach: Blood Pressure Improvement in Primary Care for African Americans

Ameling et al. (2014) researched approaches for enhancing and sustaining interventions for African Americans with uncontrolled hypertension in an urban clinical practice in Baltimore, Maryland. Ameling et al. (2014) utilized the Achieving Blood Pressure Control Together study (ACT) study, which is part of the Johns Hopkins Center to Eliminate Cardiovascular Health Disparities. They also implemented theoretical approaches, such as community-based participatory research and science frameworks to adapt behavioral interventions for use in people with uncontrolled hypertension.

According to Ameling et al. (2014), these two principles have been recommended for development of interventions that effectively address health care disparities. Ameling et al. (2014) looked at a comparison of how effective patient-centered behavioral self-management interventions would improve hypertension control in urbanized African Americans who are receiving primary care.

The authors believed that their approach of adapting the ACT study may have several advantages due to the engagement of different stakeholders in patients' care (for example, "patients and their families, health care payers, clinicians, staff and community members") (p. 132).

Furthermore, Ameling et al. (2014) stated that the methodologies they utilized to adapt intervention for blacks "could improve interventions' translation to real clinical practice settings and enhance interventions' sustained effectiveness" (p. 132). Also, their approach showed many intervention modifications to improve possible effectiveness of hypertension self-management in this specific group. Nevertheless, the authors emphasized that the effectiveness of their adaptions will not be known until their trial is completed.

Utilization of Community Settings for Lifestyle Interventions

Health promotion interventions can improve health status of people and their communities. This is especially so in countries, states and geographic areas with high prevalence of chronic diseases, for example, hypertension. Health promotion strategies such as health education can be beneficial. The implementation of health teaching in churches, community centers, or any facility or environment where people are gathered for a common purpose creates a social environment for health education programs. The implementation of evidence-based health promotion programs has been documented to possibly improve health of people in the population when these interventions are put in place in communities (Allicok et al., 2013).

Church-based settings can facilitate the implementation of lifestyle interventions, such as education to increase knowledge and awareness of healthy lifestyle behaviors. For instance, Tussing-Humphreys, Thomson, Mayo and Edmond (2013) studied 20 African American adults over 18 years old from 2010 to 2011. The purpose was to assess whether a 6-month church-based diet and physical activity intervention would be effective in improving diet quality and increase physical activity in this population living in the Lower Mississippi Delta region. Researchers obtained subjects' baseline data from July to October 2010 and post-intervention data from February to May 2011.

Tussing-Humphreys et al. (2013) reported that diseases such as hypertension, obesity and diabetes are at the epidemic stage in people residing in the rural Lower Mississippi Delta region of Mississippi. They believed that poor diet and low levels of physical activity among people in this geographic area are probably contributing factors for elevated prevalence of disease. The present clinical policy was developed from the Joint National Committee on Prevention, Detection, Evaluation, and Treatment of High Blood Pressure (JNC7). This policy suggested six self-care activities people with high blood pressure should perform: "adhering to antihypertensive medication regimens, maintaining or losing weight, following a low-salt diet, limiting alcohol, engaging in regular physical activity and eliminating tobacco use" (Warren-Findlow et al., 2012, p. 15).

This Delta Body and Soul intervention (DBS) originated from the original Body and Soul program. However, Tussing-Humphreys et al. (2013) utilized some parts of the original Body and Soul program and also made several changes to the original for their study. Churches that took part were assigned to either intervention or control. Members of the church committee were assigned specific tasks for the intervention and control groups.

For the intervention, subjects received monthly education regarding increasing consumption of fruits, vegetables, whole grains, and low-fat dairy foods, and lowering intake of solid fats, added sugars and sodium. Subjects also obtained instruction regarding adequate portion sizes and the health benefits of eating the specified food at the dietary sessions. One education event was geared towards benefits of physical activity, and strategies for overcoming physical inactivity.

Additionally, subjects obtained written information regarding the six self-care lessons, healthy recipes, and other tips on nutrition, chronic disease prevention and physical activity. These subjects also received monthly educational newsletters including information on physical activity and nutrition. Also included in the newsletters were testimonials from church members regarding the changes they made in their diet and physical activity. The control study subjects received bimonthly newsletters with information related to colds, influenza, food safety and stress reduction.

The result of the study showed significant improvement, but this was notable only in some components of diet quality in both the intervention and control groups. According to the authors, this signifies a lack of intervention effect. It was also shown that subjects in the intervention group showed increased aerobic physical activity, strength, and flexibility. But this was not observed in the control group.

It is the authors' belief that the lack of dietary intervention effect may be attributed to the subjects' level of participation. It is important to note that those in the high-participation interventions subgroup showed significant improvement in both the total and six components of diet quality. This improvement was not seen in the control group, except for whole fruits and total scores, nor in the low-participation subgroup. The findings showed improvement with whole fruits, total vegetables, dark green and orange vegetables and legumes, and whole grains, which is reassuring, because these components were provided at the educational sessions for subjects.

This result suggested subjects made steps to change their lifestyle by including healthy food from a variety of food groups in their diet. This study's dietary finding is consistent with Allicok et al. (2013), which utilized the colon cancer screening intervention Body and Soul Program in black churches in North Carolina and Michigan from 2008 through 2010. Their study showed an increase in mean fruit and vegetable consumption from baseline to follow-up period.

Interestingly, mode of transportation was a factor in the participation of intervention activities at the end of the study. It was revealed that individuals who did not own a vehicle had difficulty attending weekly church activities and educational sessions. Those who had not participated reported reasons such as lack of transportation and the increase in gas prices in the spring of 2011. Only individuals who owned a vehicle showed improvement in vegetable intake. Lack of transportation has been reported elsewhere as a barrier for people to attend education sessions. For example, Gross et al. (2013) looked at culturally sensitive educational programs for African Americans on an antihypertensive regimen; they found that some participants had not returned to the clinic for additional education sessions and blood pressure assessment (Gross et al., 2013).

"Resources in high-affluence communities, particularly access to healthy food, health care services, and physical activity opportunities, may allow economically disadvantaged residents to adopt a healthy lifestyle"(Abeyta, Tuitt, Byers, & Sauaia, 2012, p. 2). The authors concluded that for programs to be successful, people must be able to attend educational sessions and have access to transportation.

The result of the study suggests that education can help to improve lifestyle behaviors in some people if they are provided with educational tools, support and encouragement. The support will probably increase their motivation to follow through with lifestyle modifications. Written material or educational sessions may also increase awareness and understanding about the benefits of healthy foods choices and physical activity. These measures play a significant role in improving the health status of people with a chronic condition.

Church Interventions to Promote Lifestyle Changes

According to Powell-Wiley et al. (2012), cardiovascular risk factors (CVRF), such as hypertension, hyperlipidemia, diabetes and obesity, are more pronounced in African Americans, resulting in high burden of cardiovascular disease (CVD) in this group. The authors believe that if people engage in physical activity and change their diets, CVRFs can substantially improve, thus preventing CVD.

A cross-sectional analysis compared baseline data from all GoodNEWs trial subjects and Dallas County African Americans. In this study, Powell-Wiley et al. (2012) compared demographics, anthropometrics and CVRF prevalence, awareness, treatment and control between subjects in the GoodNEWs trial with age- and sex-matched African Americans in Dallas County. For this comparison, data was obtained from the Dallas Heart Study.

The GoodNEWs trial focused on interventions to promote lifestyle changes in mostly African American churches in Dallas, Texas, while the Dallas Heart Study data consisted of a multiethnic, population-based sample of Dallas County residents. The authors also evaluated whether there was an association between frequency of church attendance and CVRFs in the Dallas Heart Study group to get a better understanding of the association between church attendance and CVRFs in the GoodNEWs trial. Subjects in 20 African American churches in Dallas participated in the GoodNEWs study.

The study showed that GoodNEWs subjects were a higher-risk population with a higher prevalence of obesity, including higher obesity-related CVRFs. For example, GoodNEWs subjects were more likely to have diabetes, low levels of high-density lipoproteins (HDL), and high triglycerides when compared to blacks of similar age and gender in Dallas County. Even though GoodNEWs subjects' obesity rates were higher, they tended to exercise more, smoked less, and would seek pharmacological treatment for the control of CVRFs; their blood pressures were controlled compared to the general population. Most importantly, the GoodNEWs subjects' level of education was higher compared to the general population.

Dallas County subjects who attended church, for example, four times or more per month, had higher BMIs and waist circumferences than less frequent church goers. The prevalence of obesity was associated with subjects who went to church more frequently, that is, more than four times a month.

These findings regarding the GoodNEWs African American population who go to church frequently were supported by analysis of the Dallas Heart Study population, which revealed that more frequent church attendance is linked with obesity and decreased probability of smoking. It is the authors' belief that their findings highlighted the potential role of African American churches, where community-based interventions can be implemented.

Moreover, they believed that GoodNEWs church-based interventions, such as weight loss, could be beneficial for secondary prevention and treatment of CVRFs in blacks. Because GoodNEWs subjects showed more interest and motivation in changing their lifestyle by exercising than Dallas Heart Study subjects, Powell-Wiley and others (2012) concluded that the GoodNEWs subjects may need education about exercise to assist with weight reduction, improving risk factors of CVD, and diet. However, the authors strongly suggested that based on the result of their study, the GoodNEWs program should be targeting obesity by addressing lifestyle modifications, instead of improving awareness, treatment and control of diabetes, hypertension and hyperlipidemia.

Dietary Supplements for Hypertension

According to Woolf and Bisognano (2011), lifestyle modification is still an important aspect for hypertension management, even though there are many pharmaceutical choices. They also suggest dietary supplements for management of hypertension.

According to Woolf and Bisognano (2011), some dietary supplements, such as potassium, calcium, vitamin D, folate, fish oil, garlic, and fruit and vegetable extracts, have been found to decrease blood pressure. Woolf and Bisognano (2011) stated that potassium supplementation appears to lower systolic blood pressure on a magnitude of 3 to 12 mm Hg; dietary potassium increases may have similar benefits to supplementation. In terms of calcium, supplementation results in only mild blood pressure reduction. It is the authors' belief that calcium supplementation would only benefit those with low baseline dietary consumption of calcium.

Hypertensive people are more likely than controls to have lower vitamin D levels. The supplementation of vitamin D results in systolic blood pressure reduction of approximately 2.4 mm Hg but has no effect on diastolic blood pressure.

Woolf and Bisognano (2011) pointed to various studies showing that high dosages of fish oil supplement led to small but significant reductions in blood pressures, for example, a systolic reduction of 2 to 3 mm Hg. Even though garlic extract may lower blood pressure, and studies show decreases in systolic blood pressure, the effectiveness of garlic remains to be seen. Most importantly, the DASH diet, with the combination of fruits, vegetables, and lower saturated and total fats, has proved to lower blood pressure (Woolf and Bisognano, 2011).

Although it has been shown that some supplements tend to lower blood pressure, it is important that people consult their doctors before taking any dietary supplements. A diet that consists of foods from all groups (grains, vegetables, protein, fruit, and low-fat dairy) is important for everyone, with hypertension or not. But, people with hypertension need to be more vigilant with regard to their food intake. The approach to any intervention, whether it is dietary modification or pharmaceutical, is adherence for blood pressure improvement and effectiveness. Hypertensive people should pay special attention to their daily salt intake and the types of food they purchase to eat. Similarly, people with hypertension should build exercise in their daily routine. Hypertensive people should make an effort to be in compliance with their diet, whether individually or otherwise developed, to help control their blood pressure.

Appendix 1 provides an example of a seven-day sample menu plan. It was independently developed for an individual with hypertension. It is not intended to replace the medication prescribed for hypertension; instead, it serves to supplement medication. It is recommended that people with hypertension and those with allergies consult their doctors before starting or changing their diets.

Physical Activity for Hypertension Management

Nead et al. (2013) define the walking impairment questionnaire (WIQ) as "a subjective measure of patient-perceived walking performance" (p. 255). The authors stated that even though the WIQ was implemented for people with peripheral arterial disease (PAD), objective walking ability, which is the predictor of clinical outcomes, can be extended beyond people with PAD. The researchers pointed to the "6 minute walking test that has been shown to predict future mortality in patients with both congestive heart failure and pulmonary hypertension" (p. 255). Furthermore, the long-distance corridor walk is a component of the 60 minute walking test, and reduced gait speed has been linked to deaths and future cardiovascular disease in older adults residing in community dwellings. As a result, Nead et al. (2013) believed that subjective measures of walking ability, such as the WIQ tool, may be valuable predictors of risk even if individuals are free of PAD.

Nead et al. (2013) conducted the Genetic Determinants of Peripheral Arterial Disease (GenePAD) study on 1417 subjects of diverse ethnic groups (white, black, Hispanic, Asian, and other). The researchers tested whether lower WIQ category scores had an association with future all-cause and cardiovascular mortality in individuals with PAD, and whether the test could be extended to people without PAD. They also examined whether the WIQ could improve the present clinical tools and provide an independent improvement in capacity, discriminatory ability, and net reclassification parameters of established cardiovascular risk prediction models in an at-risk cohort.

For this study, subjects completed the WIQ at baseline. The WIQ consisted of three categories. These were assessing walking distance, stair climbing and walking speed. The baseline assessment of these categories was carried out on subjects who were having coronary angiography procedures. Subjects provided degree of difficulty for each activity category. The responses ranged from zero, meaning they were unable, to four, which indicated no difficulty. Subjects were required to answer questions, estimating ranges for each of the activities. For example, "walking distance ranged from walking indoors to walking 1500 feet, stair climbing was from climbing one flight of stairs to climbing three flights of stairs, while walking speed ranged from walking one block slowly to jogging one block." The questions in each category were weighted based on the difficulty subjects encountered performing them.

The results showed a significant connection in subjects without PAD. Also, there was no significant difference based on subjects' PAD condition. Lower WIQ distance, stair climbing and speed scores were shown to independently predict future all-cause and cardiovascular deaths in subjects who were high-risk. Further, those who had reported deficit scores of less than 100 percent in walking distance, stair climbing, and walking speed were linked to a significant increased risk of mortality from any cause. Nevertheless, the scores revealed in each of the three categories pointed to a significant "improved risk discrimination and reclassification for all-cause and cardiovascular mortality over the baseline model of cardiovascular risk factors and the model of SCORE risk variables" (p. 259).

The authors believe that the WIQ probably will be beneficial clinically, because this tool may be able to evaluate the risk of death in the future in those people who are at high risk for cardiovascular events despite PAD status. It is important to note that of the WIQ categories, the scores in stair climbing were frequently the strongest predictor of risk. More importantly, the follow-up after a median of 5 years showed that 172 subjects out of 1417 died. Of 172, 47 deaths were due to cardiovascular causes, for example, myocardial infarction, cardiac arrest, stroke, heart failure or aneurysm rupture. According to the researchers, their findings also proved that WIQ improves the accuracy of risk models.

Stamler et al. (2013) report that black African Americans' blood pressure is higher compared to non-Hispanic white Americans, and there is no explanation for differences in etiopathogenesis. They believe that multiple black to white differences may exist in food or nutrient intake and urinary metabolites, causing higher blood pressure in blacks. Stamler et al. (2013) utilized INTERMAP data to examine 369 African Americans and 1190 non-Hispanic white Americans; all were women and men 40 to 59 years of age, recruited from a random U.S. population sample in the online-only data supplement. Subjects completed questionnaires, had their height and weight measured, blood pressure measured on eight occasions, and 24-hour urine collected twice; data included 24-hour dietary recalls.

The study showed that the higher systolic and diastolic blood pressure in African Americans was a result of consumption of multiple less-favorable nutrients. African American intake of foods and nutrients possibly favorable to blood pressure was lower, for example, "raw vegetables, fresh fruits, vegetable protein, total grains, potassium, glycine, magnesium, fiber," to name a few. Additionally, average BMI was higher for black women, as were their rates of obesity compared to those of white women.

Further, African Americans' intake of foods and nutrients that would possibly have adverse effects on blood pressure was higher. It was shown that this group consumed "higher processed meats, pork, eggs, sugar-sweetened beverages, total sugars and dietary cholesterol."

Blacks' intake was favorable for only a few foods and nutrients possibly favorable to blood pressure. These were "fish/fish roe/shellfish, poultry, polyunsaturated fatty acids, polyunsaturated fatty acid ratio, and oleic acid."

In terms of urinary metabolites, many were significantly higher in black subjects than white subjects, for example, creatinine (increased levels are an indicator of kidney function), 3-hydroxyisovalerate, *N*-acetyl neuraminic acid, and others. In whites, there were four significantly higher metabolites: "trimethylamine, N-methyl nicotinic acid, hippurate and succinate."

Stamler et al. (2013) stated that the INTERMAP findings are reproducible, etiologically significant, and illustrate the need for African Americans to improve their nutritional status. They believed that this specific group would benefit from the DASH diet recommendations to prevent and control adverse blood pressure. They also emphasized the need for blacks, especially women, to decrease BMI, because higher BMI has been linked to higher blood pressure.

It is crucial for African Americans with hypertension to institute lifestyle changes by modifying their diet. They should include in their diets foods and nutrients that would produce a positive effect on blood pressure levels. In combination, diet and physical activity would probably have a major impact on blood pressure control, management, and prevalence in African American populations.

Hypertension: Gait Slowing in Older Adults

Physical activity is important for people with hypertension. This intervention can help with physical functional abilities and possibly decrease disability as people age.

For instance, the Cardiovascular Health Study (CHS), a multicenter population-based longitudinal study of risk factors for cardiovascular disease in older adults, examined gait slowing in relation to blood pressure (Rosano et al., 2011). The study consisted of 2733 parent cohort subjects and a selected group of 643 subjects, both black and white, male and female, of which 15 percent were black.

For subjects to be included in the study, they had a baseline magnetic resonance imaging (MRI) scan, and their mobility and systolic blood pressure measured, and no self-reported disability from 1992 to 1994. They were also required to have at least one follow-up gait speed measurement from 1997 to 1999 and again in 2005 to 2006. In addition, a second MRI during 1997 to 1999 was required.

Rosano et al. (2011) looked at whether hypertension was associated with decline in gait speed, whether it was significant in older adult subjects who were well-functioning, and whether health-related factors, for example, brain, kidney and heart function, could provide the reason.

The study showed that hypertension lowered gait speed in well-functioning community-dwelling older adults. This was observed over a follow-up of over 14 years. Not only were significant associations observed in newly diagnosed subjects, and the previously diagnosed with uncontrolled hypertension, but also for those whose blood pressure was successfully controlled ("the previously diagnosed and controlled hypertension group"). Nevertheless, the association between the subjects' being exposed to high blood pressure and their decline in gait speed was not independent of, nor was it reduced by, other risk factors that contribute to slower gait.

These included measures and conditions that are believed to be associated with hypertension and probably components of gait slowing, such as integrity of the brain, kidney, and heart, as well as stroke and dementia incidents.

Moreover, the health-related measurements did not provide a reason for these associations. The authors stated that their study focus looked at the pathway that links hypertension with gait slowing through vascular-related brain abnormalities. However, they also believed that exposure to high blood pressure probably has an incubation period of greater than 5 years before it would establish a solid change in end organs, namely kidney, heart, and brain. This they thought was the reason for the accelerated gait slowing in the group of subjects who were newly diagnosed with hypertension, which was independent of five-year white matter hyperintensity progression.

The findings also revealed a significant association with high systolic blood pressure and the rate of gait speed decline in the selected (643) subjects, and it was similar for the 2733 parent cohort subjects.

The subjects with exposure to high blood pressure, previously diagnosed hypertensives that were both controlled and uncontrolled, had a significantly faster rate of gait speed decline compared to those without hypertension and whose baseline blood pressure measurement was less than 140/90 mm Hg.

The study showed that high blood pressure plays a role in physical functional decline in older people. Policy planners should consider implementing interventions for older people in community settings to increase physical activities, thus promoting health, well-being, and graceful aging. Barriers to adherence for hypertension treatment have been reported in other research. For example, Gross et al. (2013) revealed that African American people older than 65 years had not taken part in a regular exercise program. And older females had voiced concerns about their safety walking in their neighborhood. The reasons provided by the majority were either affordability (to join a gym or fitness club) or, if they had the desire to walk in the mall, lack of transportation.

Exercise is equally as important as dietary measures in terms of lifestyle modification for people living with hypertension. Any physical activity could be an effective method for controlling and improving blood pressure. Bell, Lutsey,

Windham and Folsom (2013) rightly stated that "some physical activity is better than none" (p. 907).

A survey by Wexler et al. (2008) was carried out on 244 patients who received health care within the Ohio State University primary care practice-based research network. Of these patients, 57 percent were women, 51 percent white and 43 percent African Americans. Patients were diagnosed with hypertension. Questions on the survey were used to determine basic demographics and stage of change for diet and exercise in hypertensive patients. The stage-of-change question was "Have you changed your diet (reduced sodium, decreased alcohol, lowered fat) or exercise habits to help lower your blood pressure?" They were instructed to choose one of five options. The patients were also asked to report preferred lifestyle choice. These were "exercise, weight loss, reduced salt, increased fruits and vegetables, or moderation of alcohol" (p. 359).

The survey findings showed that most white patients were more likely to exercise, but this was not shown in African American patients. Black subjects chose option 3, which states "no, but I intended to exercise in the next 30 days" (p. 359). Nonetheless, patients chose exercise as their preferred lifestyle choice over reduced salt, weight loss, and moderation of alcohol intake.

The authors pointed to other studies that reported barriers to exercise and desired lifestyle behaviors in patients of lower socioeconomic statuses, higher neighborhood crime rates, lower social support and those with baseline general poor health. Despite these disparities, Wexler et al. (2008) stated that there was no difference in education between African Americans and whites; similar percentages of both groups graduated from high school or college. The vast difference was seen in income levels between whites and African Americans. The yearly income for 35 percent of African American patients was less than $25,000, while for whites, only 23 percent were in the same income group. The authors believed that based on their findings, low income is positively linked with African Americans' thinking about exercise.

A cross-sectional study of a large group comprised of equal gender numbers and cultural background may be necessary. The study should examine whether thinking about exercise is strongly associated with performing it more frequently and whether socioeconomic condition is a factor. People need to continually be reminded about the consequences of consuming too much salt. They should also be educated about the benefits of a low-salt diet in combination with exercise for effective control and management of hypertension.

It is important for community program educators to focus not only on interventions but also consider the cultural needs of people. Given that dietary needs may differ based on cultural background, food preparation in the household, and what people find enticing, a better understanding of these factors may motivate people, increasing knowledge and adherence. Some people may find it difficult to abstain from certain foods because they find it too restricting to do so. For example, food without salt may not have the same taste for one group while for other groups there is no difference. Similarly, lifestyle modifications may be effective for some people and not for others. However, it is still worthwhile to implement lifestyle modifications because for many people with high blood pressure, the need for medication will be decreased (Kolasa et al., 2012), although "experiencing the consequences of dietary change is a much longer process" (p. 181).

According to Bier et al. (2008), people who develop dietary guidelines should consider consumer health goals, for example, preventing common chronic disease. Popular views about health may inspire consumers to follow dietary guidance and should be included in guidance messages (Bier et al., 2008).

One approach is to abstain from unhealthy foods but allow some unhealthy foods in moderation so that people can enjoy their meals and meet their nutritional health needs without jeopardizing their blood pressure levels. Most of all, educators should be well equipped in nutrition and food preparation and be knowledgeable about the culture of people they are counseling. These measures will give educators an insight to provide effective counseling about dietary needs. This is especially so for people with low incomes, because some people may have limited choices when purchasing food. Educators can assist this group by educating them about food substitutes with similar nutritional value and low salt content. Educators should also try to encourage people and provide support to increase their motivation. People may be more adherent if others show that they care about their well-being. For example, Gross et al. (2013) showed that African Americans who agreed to a follow-up telephone call in week three following a completed culturally sensitive educational program to improve adherence in anti-hypertension regimen liked the individualized attention they received.

Nutritional Intake and Physical Activity as Cardiovascular Risk Factors

Research continually points to hypertension as one of the major risk factors for cardiovascular disease. In the same way, both hypertension and prehypertension have been linked to other cardiovascular risk factors, for example, obesity and hypercholesterolemia. Women are at risk for hypertension as their age increases, and it is believed to be more common in women after 59 years of age than in men (Hageman, Carol, Pullen, Noble, & Boeckher, 2010).

The Wellness for Women project was conducted by Hageman et al. (2010). This community-based clinical trial was conducted by an interdisciplinary team of nurses, a physical therapist and a dietician. The team goal was to promote healthy eating and physical activity among rural Midwestern women. Subjects were 225 rural women ages 50 to 69 enrolled in a healthy eating and activity clinical trial. The study looked at whether participants who had prehypertension or hypertension when they enrolled would also have other cardiovascular risk factors, namely low fitness or dyslipidemia. To determine this, the authors looked at participants' cardiovascular health histories, medication usage, fitness, lipids, and blood pressure readings, identifying participants as normotensive, prehypertensive, or hypertensive. This was important to examine because most participants' enrolled blood pressures were either in the prehypertensive or hypertensive ranges. As such, Hageman et al. (2010) expected that a high prevalence of cardiovascular disease, medication usage, dyslipidemia, and lower fitness would be seen in these participants. It is important to note that for this study, participants completed a questionnaire in which they self-reported their demographics and health histories.

In comparison to the normotensive group, a high prevalence of self-reported cardiovascular disease and of non-optimal values of HDL cholesterol, triglycerides and estimated cardiovascular fitness was documented in the hypertensive group. Whereas, in the normotensive blood pressure group, other cardiovascular risks factors were prevalent, for example, 61 percent of normotensive subjects were overweight or obese. The majority had elevated low-density lipoprotein (LDL) cholesterol, and low fitness was observed.

It was also shown that participants who had prehypertension and hypertension were likely to be taking medications to decrease their lipids. Many were also overweight or obese, their walking was slower, and their cardiorespiratory fitness was lower compared to participants with normotensive blood pressure readings.

In terms of the 1-mile walk test and VO_2 max, participants in both the prehypertensive and hypertensive groups had abnormal distributions and the variance was larger compared to the normotensive group of participants. Most importantly, participants with either prehypertensive or hypertensive blood pressures percentages were likely to have low estimated cardiovascular fitness. When walking speed is measured, 50-year-old participants should be able to walk at a rate of at least 3 miles in an hour, but an alarming 72 percent of participants walked one mile. Also, 15 women who were obese walked too slowly to estimate VO_2 max.

The study also revealed that the prevalence of prehypertension (52.2 percent) and hypertension (20.8 percent) was higher compared to findings in similar rural Midwestern populations with prehypertension of 33.1 percent and hypertension of 10.3 percent. The authors also compared their findings of cholesterol results to the national data of non-Hispanic white women of age 20 years. Total cholesterol prevalence was high, over 200 mg/dL for this wellness study (51.6 percent), while in national data for non-Hispanic white women it was only 47.7 percent.

Hageman et al. (2010) believe that routine assessment and screening of blood pressure and other vital signs should be performed by clinicians. Given the high prevalence of prehypertension and hypertension among the enrolled participants, many may not have been aware of their condition. Most of all they reported that when patients' blood pressure readings reveal prehypertension or hypertension, it is important that these patients are provided with additional counseling, a referral should be made, and the counseling should be focused on foreseeable cardiovascular risk factors.

Studies show that stress management effectively reduces systolic blood pressure. Dusek et al. (2008) stated that after the age of 60, there is a tendency toward increases in systolic blood pressure, whereas diastolic blood pressure is likely to decrease; 65 to 75 percent of elderly people with hypertension have "isolated systolic hypertension." According to the author, systolic hypertension is defined as systolic blood pressure higher than 140 mm Hg and diastolic pressure less than 90 mm Hg. Dusek and his colleagues pointed to the economic impact this blood pressure level will have on the American people and the foreseeable health condition in the twenty-first century although the JNC8 recommendations take the normal rise in systolic pressure by the elderly into account.

Dusek et al. (2008) reports that stress management techniques that bring about the relaxation response are safe for the treatment of essential hypertension. He conducted a randomized trial comparing eight weeks of stress management, specifically relaxation response training versus lifestyle modification, among 61 subjects in the relaxation response group and 61 subjects in the control group. Subjects were 55 years and over, diagnosed with systolic hypertension. The purpose of the study was to determine whether eight weeks of training in eliciting the relaxation response versus eight weeks of lifestyle modification would decrease systolic blood pressure in elderly subjects with systolic hypertension.

This study showed that in elderly subjects who had eight weeks of stress management training by elicitation of the relaxation response and lifestyle modification, systolic blood pressure was decreased more than 9 mm Hg. In the relaxation group the decrease was 9.4 mm Hg and in the control group, 8.8 mm Hg. According to Dusek, the findings are comparable with other studies of people with systolic hypertension who followed eight weeks on the DASH diet, resulting in a 11.8 mm Hg decrease in systolic blood pressure. They further reported that their study and the DASH trial "are the only nonpharmacologic interventions that consistently and significantly reduce systolic blood pressure in hard-to treat elderly adults with systolic hypertension" (p. 135). The authors report that their study findings are likely to be generalized. This is because 36 subjects, equivalent to 30 percent, were 70 to 79 years of age while five (4 percent) were greater than 80 years of age. It is important to note that the average age of subjects was 67 years. Of greater interest, the authors found that systolic blood pressure was decreased in both the relaxation response group and control group. This reduction was similar and greater than expected. Also, it was demonstrated that two-thirds of study subjects had reacted to nonpharmacologic therapy.

Subjects who obtained a systolic reading of less than 140 mm Hg and a decrease of 5 mm Hg or better in systolic blood pressure met the eligibility criteria for an additional eight weeks of training with supervised medication elimination. The result also showed that a high proportion of subjects in the relaxation response group had at least one of their blood pressure medications successfully removed, more than those in the control group. It was also shown that the removal of antihypertensive medications in the groups was not a concern.

Dusek et al. (2008) stated that a decrease in systolic blood pressure of 5 mm Hg reduces early death by 7 percent and stroke risk by 30 percent. In conclusion, the authors reported that the result of their study has clinical impact. The study suggests a need to control systolic blood pressure levels especially in elderly people, because of the rising rate of elderly people with hypertension. Treatment interventions, whether medication or nonpharmalogic measures, could help decrease illnesses and death attributed to higher systolic blood pressure levels.

Self-Efficacy and Self-Care Management for Hypertension

"Failure to achieve chronic disease treatment goals arises from both patient treatment nonadherence and inadequate treatment intensification" (Crowley et al., 2013, p. 179). Given that hypertension is a chronic disease, it is important that people carry out different self-care behaviors to manage this condition. The psychosocial concept of self-efficacy has been linked to patients' ability to manage chronic disease (Warren- Findlow et al., 2012).

Warren-Findlow et al. (2012) studied 190 African Americans age 22 to 88 years; more than half were 50 years of age and over, and almost 70 percent were female with hypertension. Subjects were interviewed about their self-efficacy and self-care activities for their hypertension. The authors examined the association between self-efficacy to manage hypertension and six clinical prescribed self-care behaviors, such as medication adherence, low-salt diet adherence, physical activity adherence, smoking cessation, alcohol abstinence, and weight management adherence. The Caring for Hypertension in African American Families study was carried out during September 2008 to August 2010 at the University of North Carolina at Charlotte.

The results showed that more than half of African American subjects had good self-efficacy to manage their hypertension. This was reported in five of the six hypertension self-care activities. Subjects with good self-efficacy had better rates of adherence to medication, maintenance of low-salt diet techniques (64 percent), performance of physical activity (27 percent), not smoking (10 percent), and following good weight management strategies (63 percent).

However, better self-efficacy had no association with refraining from alcohol. This result had led Warren-Findlow et al. (2012) to alert health providers to increase awareness by informing patients about alcohol intake and its effect on blood pressure management.

It is important to note that most of the adult subjects in this study were younger with hypertension. The education and income levels indicate that subjects were middle class.

Overall, the study showed that this population was knowledgeable about self-efficacy for blood pressure management. The result is promising for the application of self-improvement for hypertension management because subjects showed a vested interest in their health. Still, African American people with hypertension need to be persistent in finding different strategies to decrease their weight, because most of these subjects were considered clinically overweight or obese. Also, they should continually be encouraged to increase their motivational levels.

A Review of Patient-Tailored Self-Management for Blood Pressure

According to Park, Chang, Kim and Kwak (2012), older patients with hypertension in nursing homes in Korea require a tailored self-management plan along with a lifestyle approach. They stated that it may be questioned why subjects need this strategy when staff are available at the facility. But the authors believe that such an approach is needed because poor self-management is frequent in this population once they are placed in a nursing home. This is because these residents previously relied on family members to assist them with the care of their hypertension in their homes, but once they are placed in a nursing home, the support is no longer available.

Despite an extension of health insurance coverage to assist in nursing home care, following an increase in patients in Korean nursing homes, qualified staff who should be caring for these patients has not increased; as a result there is a cause for concern regarding the quality of care patients receive in the facilities.

Park et al. (2012) have pointed to the potential benefits for patient-tailored self-management intervention with a lifestyle approach for blood pressure control. First, this approach would be beneficial to both residents and staff in the facility. Secondly, if the nursing home accepts this approach, residents may be empowered to adjust to the new environment and become more engaged in their care. Also, for residents who are given the opportunity to participate in the care of their hypertension, blood pressure could be controlled and their capability of self-care could increase.

Definition of Self-Management

Radhakrishnan (2011) defines self-management as "the individual's ability to manage the symptoms, treatment, physical and psychosocial consequences and lifestyle changes inherent in living with a long term disorder" (p. 497).

Self-Management for Blood Pressure Control

Park, Chang, Kim and Kwak (2012) evaluated the efficacy of patient-tailored self-management intervention with lifestyle modification for primary blood pressure control in older adults with hypertension residing in a nursing home. Short-term effects of the intervention on self-care behavior, exercise, self-efficacy, and medication adherence were also evaluated.

This intervention study consisted of a total of 47 residents assigned to two groups. The control group consisted of 24 and the intervention group 23 residents. To increase self-management, the intervention group residents were provided with health education and tailored individual counseling for eight weeks.

The results showed that residents were taking blood pressure medication for approximately 11 years. Thirty-six residents did not require assistance with taking medication, while 16 required assistance. It is important to note that the majority of residents were female (72 percent), one-third were married, and their average age was 77.4 years.

The findings revealed that patient-tailored self-management intervention reduced residents' blood pressure. It was shown that there was significant interaction of patient-tailored self-management in both the intervention and control group from baseline to eight weeks later in both systolic and diastolic blood pressures. Also, after eight weeks, systolic and diastolic blood pressures were lower compared to baseline blood pressure levels. However, while blood pressure was significantly decreased, the improvement was only noted in the intervention group.

In terms of self-care behavior, exercise self-efficacy, and medication adherence, the patient-tailored self-management in the intervention group showed a significant improvement in all secondary outcomes. But this was not shown in medication adherence in either the intervention or comparison (control) group. It was also revealed that self-care behavior had improved significantly from baseline to eight weeks later. This was observed in residents in the intervention group, with an increase of 13.7 points, whereas there was a decrease of 3.4 points in the comparison group. Both self-care behavior and exercise efficacy were further decreased from baseline to eight weeks later in those in the comparison group.

The authors stated that three intervention effects came into play from their findings. For instance, the self-management intervention had considered the residents' needs and preferences, for example, their concerns regarding self-management and the challenges of the environment; the end result was a greater reduction in blood pressure. According to Radhakrishnan (2011), tailored interventions are considered a combination of patient-centered and patient-empowerment approaches. This means the interventions are always tailored to the person, based on the first assessment.

The study shows that educational materials and individual counseling tailored to individual needs are potentially effective methods for decreasing blood pressure regardless of the setting. Moreover, "the self-efficacy of nursing home residents may allow them to be more responsive to lifestyle changes for hypertension management" (Park et al., 2012, p. 718). This study is consistent with Gross et al. (2013), where 100 percent of African Americans had increased knowledge regarding hypertension treatment after education sessions.

Tailored Interventions' Effectiveness: Self-Management Behaviors for Chronic Diseases

In a similar study by Radhakrishnan (2011), the author evaluated the effectiveness of tailored interventions on self-management behaviors in people with heart disease, hypertension and type 2 diabetes. Radhakrishnan (2011) reports that because differences exist between individuals, successful self-management for the long term is more likely when the delivery of interventions is tailored to the specific individual.

In this study, the author reviewed randomized control trials published between 2001 and 2010 using several databases, such as Pubmed, CINAHL, PsychInfor, ERIC, ASP, WOS and SSA. Reference lists from relevant articles were also looked at. The specific search term criteria were "tailored intervention(s)" and "self-management for chronic diseases." Radhakrishnan (2011) reviewed ten studies for the medical literature review. Included in the review was a comparison of a tailored intervention against the usual care or alternative forms of interventions that promote self-management. A combination of tailored interventions was used, such as initial in-person counseling followed with telephone calls. This was used in five out of the ten studies.

The team consisted of multiple providers that delivered tailored interventions. For example, nurses delivered the tailored interventions either alone or as part of the team for four of the nine studies that included the study on home blood pressure monitoring. After extensive training, lay educators or counselors delivered tailored interventions to improve diabetic retinopathy screening. Other providers of interventions included primary care physicians or general practitioners (three studies), and nurse practitioners (one study). Another study utilized postal mail over health care providers to deliver intervention, while in one study a research psychologist delivered tailored intervention at a diabetes center.

The assessment of quality for the ten randomized control trials showed high scores for several studies, for example, the Bosworth et al. (2011) study about home blood pressure monitoring, which included the subjects' eligibility criterion of having hypertension for at least one year. In contrast, the lowest score was for the 2008 Dutton et al. study which tested tailored interventions for increasing physical activity in subjects with type 2 diabetes (as cited in Radhakrishnan, 2011).

Blood pressure improvement was better in studies that employed a combination of tailored interventions with home blood pressure monitoring, for instance, as in Bosworth et al. (2011). However, tailored interventions were minimally successful for improving self-management behaviors in subjects with long-term conditions. There was no association between the length or amount of tailored interventions and the aimed results in the ten studies reviewed. Cost and resource utilization in the development and implementation was reported as pitfalls in two of the studies; for example, Bosworth et al. (2011) reported that tailored interventions were expensive to put in place. Nevertheless in one study, "patients reported that periodic support from their physician was the most important component of the tailored intervention" (p. 506).

Overall, this study did not show that tailored interventions had an effect on self-management activities such as adhering to medication regime, self-monitoring, exercise, smoking or dietary control. But tailored interventions were shown to have success in self-management behaviors such as subjects' consumption of dietary fat, physical activity levels, and screening.

Radhakrishnan (2011) concluded that although tailored interventions are one of the several strategies recommended to guide nurses in the support of people with long-term conditions, the effectiveness of this strategy in improving self-management remains inconclusive when considering the utilization of resources and cost. Additionally, this strategy may not be as effective as the standard care interventions for improving self-management behaviors in those afflicted with chronic conditions.

Cultural attitudes and beliefs may play a role in self-care behaviors in people with hypertension. In a study examining African American attitudes and beliefs regarding preventive behaviors for hypertension, Peters et al. (2006) utilized the theory of planned behavior as a guide to gather information from subjects. The five focus groups included three women's groups and two men's groups, for a total of 34 African American subjects from 27 to 60 years old.

According to the authors, the theory of planned behavior has been used in abundant studies to explain and predict how human beings behave. It is the authors' belief that this theory can help in addressing the knowledge gap. This can be done by implementing a framework that would seek attitudes and beliefs that blacks tend to hold that influence their participation level in hypertension prevention behaviors.

In terms of hypertension preventative beliefs, the findings showed that culturally prescribed norms regarding diet and food preparation were viewed as the cause for subjects' hypertension. Yet, not much attention was given to obesity and exercise as factors that contributed to their hypertension. The contribution of diet to blood pressure was attributed to ingredients in food, such as salt and fat, instead of weight and how weight affects blood pressure. Note that subjects in the five groups had not placed much importance on controlling their weight or increasing their physical activity as a strategy for prevention and control of their blood pressure. Subjects also believed that the "stressful lives" they lead was the reason for their hypertension. Additionally, the stressful lives were an obstacle to participate in preventive self-care. Subjects with higher socioeconomic status perceived that their stress arises from busy lives from work and commitments from their family, while those of lower socioeconomic status reported that their stress was due to lack of finances required to meet their basic needs.

Regarding the theory of planned behavior, subjects had a strong belief that they were connected to a wider African American culture that goes further than their immediate social network. It was shown that subjects' need for hypertension prevention was demonstrated in the positive attitudes they portrayed. They also understood that changing their diets, exercising more and decreasing stress would control their blood pressure.

According to Peters et al. (2006), information from their study expanded the circle involving participants' sense of "fictive kinship" or "collective identity" (Peters et al., 2006, p. 10). However, "the sub-theme of 'acting white' emerged in discussions surrounding the lack of trust in physicians" (p. 11). Although subjects believed that the involvement of a physician was necessary to control their blood pressure, their attitude toward physicians was distrust. This distrust had caused a lack of adherence to medical care plans. African American subjects talked about their personal experiences and shared familial experiences, as well as the collective experience of the Tuskegee experiment. They believed these examples were discriminatory and had molded "their attitudes towards health care and health care providers" (p. 11). Additionally, subjects believed that if they adhered to the recommended diet, weight, and activity, other African Americans would perceive them as "acting white," as if they had left their culture behind.

It was evident from subthemes that emerged within the circle of culture that test subjects encountered difficulties whenever they attempted to participate in hypertension-preventive self-care behaviors. Nevertheless, those in the focus group had voiced interest in getting professional assistance to make changes; for example, making their culturally favored foods healthier but at the same time palatable to family members. In addition to this, social networks, for instance church, were described as places of importance to subjects as a starting point for making community-level changes.

The findings suggest the need for further education and awareness, not only in the hospital setting but also in communities. Such additional knowledge will enable individuals who are providing care to this population to gain insight and better understand their attitudes and cultural beliefs. Similarly, caregivers need to understand how these values affect adherence in controlling and managing a chronic disease such as hypertension.

8

Pharmacological Management for Hypertension

When people with high blood pressure take their medications as prescribed by their health care practitioner, they are helping to control and manage their high blood pressure.

The effort to control and manage hypertension is necessary to prevent widespread illness and death due to poor blood pressure control. This is paramount because the prevalence of this disease continues to be high in some countries. For example, the prevalence of hypertension is high in the United States, with about 70 million people affected (CDC, 2015). The prevalence of this disease is also high in Taiwan (Li et al., 2012). Hypertension ranged from the ninth through twelfth-leading cause of mortality in Taiwan between 1991 and 2008. In the United States, it is "the most prevalent form of cardiovascular disease" and contributes to death (Quinones, Liang and Ye, 2012, p. 175). One-third of adult people in the United States suffer from high blood pressure. This figure is considered high and there is great need to lower it. Therefore, all efforts should be aimed at preventing and decreasing hypertension, not only in the United States but also globally.

Heart disease and stroke are serious health problems. Treating these conditions can be costly, not only for the individuals but also for the health care system. This is especially true for people living in countries with limited health care coverage or without health care insurance. Moreover, these two debilitating conditions can have devastating impacts on overall health and well-being. This is especially true when there is limited family support, people suffer from disability due to a stroke, or when there are limited funds to purchase medication to stabilize or treat their health conditions. The burden of hypertension and its related illnesses will continue to increase worldwide if this disease is not controlled.

Older age has been associated with an increase in the incidence and prevalence of high blood pressure (Munger, 2010), and because the prevalence of this condition is reported to be high in older adults, it is quickly becoming a major public health problem (Park, Kim, Jang, & Koh, 2014). For example, Munger (2010) stated that the National Health and Nutritional Examination Survey from 1999 to 2000 showed that 20.2 percent of U.S. adults 65 to 74 years of age had hypertension, compared to 21.8 percent of those 75 or older. People with hypertension are equally responsible for taking an interest in their health to decrease their chances of illness from untreated or uncontrolled blood pressure. When people take their blood pressure medication as prescribed, they are helping to control their blood pressure and prevent hypertension health complications.

According to Pasucci, Leasure, Belknap and Kodumthara (2010), nonadherence to medication cost the U.S. economy an estimated $100 billion yearly, and "persistent adherence to prescribed medication is an important cornerstone of blood pressure control" (Holt et al., 2013, p. 558). Lack of adherence to a medication regimen has been widely described as one of the factors contributing to poor blood pressure control. The challenge to effectively control and manage hypertension with medication alone poses great difficulty for both health care practitioners and some individuals. One of the reasons is that a number of people may require more than one blood pressure medication to control their blood pressure.

Park et al. (2014) state that for the most part, about 50 percent of people with hypertension refrain from taking the medication that has been prescribed for them. Consistent with Leung et al. (2012), they reported that "over half of patients do not adhere to their prescribed medication" (p. 20). For this reason, more than $100 billion has been used on hospitalizations that could have been avoided. Further, poor medication adherence and its sequelae in the clinical setting pose a challenge for providers, with an outcry needed from a lot of individuals to focus on "medication adherence as a priority in health care reform" (Leung et al., 2012, p. 20).

The CDC (2012) data analysis from the National Health and Nutrition Examination Survey from 2003 to 2010 reported that the proportion of blacks and Mexican Americans with stage one hypertension and stage two hypertension was greater than their white counterparts. Moreover, for people with stage one hypertension, medication treatment measures were significant lower in Mexican Americans than non-Hispanics. Furthermore, the CDC (2012) also reported that although there was no racial or ethnic difference among individuals with stage two hypertension in terms of treatment, less than 60 percent with this hypertension stage had medication treatment.

There are many antihypertensive medications on the market, but health care practitioners should determine the appropriate medication for people with high blood pressure. The CDC (2012) stated that clinically, it is recommended that a more extensive treatment and follow-up regimen be focused on people with stage two hypertension. This is because risk of cardiovascular death increases as blood pressure rises.

This chapter will focus on medication management for blood pressure control. Some of the major medications used to treat hypertension will be briefly covered. Research regarding pharmacological management for hypertension will also be summarized.

Hypertension and Increased Age

Managing a chronic disease like hypertension takes effort, motivation, compliance with prescribed medication, and lifestyle modification and interventions. "As age increases so does chronic illness" (Pasucci et al., 2010, p. 5). Similarly, the prevalence of hypertension tends to increase as people age (Howard et al., 2009), and it becomes more difficult to control (Wojciechowski, Papademetriou, Faselis & Fletcher, 2008). Therefore, it is vital that people with this chronic disease follow their medication regime as prescribed by their health care provider, follow-up with their doctor as required, and work toward an open patient-physician relationship.

But although some older adults with hypertension intend to adhere to their antihypertensive medication regime, many people fail to comply. According to Park et al. (2014), there is no clear cause for this. But the authors have pointed to an earlier study which examined older adults and found that memory and cognitive functions were frequently reported as reasons for missed doses.

Howard et al. (2009) stated that African Americans are disproportionately affected by this condition, and they have less-than-optimal control of their hypertension. Even though more than 30 years of evidence has shown the benefits of pharmacological therapy, African Americans' adherence to antihypertensive medication has been reported as a major barrier to blood pressure control. Additionally, their higher prevalence of hypertension is a prime cause of cardiovascular morbidity and mortality (Schoenthaler et al., 2009). According to Howard et al. (2009), there are some factors that have contributed to racial disparities in the prevalence of hypertension and control. These are diet, physical activity, health insurance and access to quality health care. Further, Schoenthaler et al. (2009) stated that "unequal treatments, the perceived quality of interpersonal communication within the patient-provider relationship is a potential mechanism for the worse health outcomes noted in minority populations" (p. 187).

Consistent Care Versus Standard Care for Blood Pressure Control Among African Americans and Whites

Howard et al. (2009) conducted a population-based, observational study describing the relationship between consistency of care and blood pressure control over a 12-year timeframe. Individuals were elderly African Americans and whites, mostly from rural areas of North Carolina.

The study showed that during the 12-year period, subjects who received consistent care or inconsistent care had greater blood pressure control than those with no standard care. Even though most subjects had consistent care, it was noted that more white subjects had consistent care. It was also shown that diastolic blood pressure was greater in African Americans than whites. But no racial differences were seen in blood pressure control over time among subjects. The majority of subjects stated that their health was either good or excellent. However, over a period of time fewer African Americans stated that their health was excellent or good. For instance, diagnosed health conditions during four waves demonstrated that a greater proportion of whites reported they had cancer, whereas a greater amount of African Americans reported they had diabetes.

African Americans more often had inconsistent care or no standard care compared to white subjects. African Americans also had more Medicaid coverage, while whites had Medigap supplemental insurance. More African Americans were cared for at public clinics while more whites had care from private practice.

Howard et al. (2009) stated that because African Americans were less likely to have private supplemental health insurance, which helped to pay money out-of-pocket, "lack of financial resources may be a barrier to hypertension management" (p. 313). Dissatisfaction with former care received may produce a lack of trust in the health care system and discourage health care-seeking behaviors. More efforts are required to decrease barriers to the accessibility of health care and low-cost medication. Also, clinicians' knowledge of hypertension treatment needs to be broadened, and they also need to stick to clinical guidelines (CDC, 2012).

Medicine

Moore, Karanja, Svetkey and Jenkins (2011) stated that there are many blood pressure medications, and the doctor will often prescribe more than one.

This is done because the doctor needs to determine which one is more beneficial for the individual. According to Chrysant et al. (2012), "monotherapy is inadequate to control blood pressure in most patients with hypertension, regardless of race, and combination therapy with two or more antihypertensive agents is required" (p. 234). In addition, combination therapy may also improve safety and tolerability of pharmacotherapy.

Forms of Medication Used for Hypertension

According to Moore et al. (2011), some high blood pressure medications are as follows:

1. Diuretics, often referred to as water pills
2. Angiotensin-converting enzyme (ACE) inhibitors
3. Beta blockers
4. Calcium channel blockers
5. Vasodilators
6. Central nervous system agents
7. Angiotensin II inhibitors

Functions of Blood Pressure Medications

- Diuretics remove excess water and salt from the body.
- ACE inhibitors interfere with how angiotensin is made.
- Beta-blockers decrease the heart rate and output of blood. This is done by blocking noradrenaline hormone at its receptor site.
- Calcium channel blockers relax blood vessels.
- Vasodilators relax blood vessel walls, thereby dilating vessels. As a result, blood pressure is decreased.
- Central nervous system agents stop the brain from sending impulses that would make blood vessels more active, thereby narrowing them and increasing blood pressure.
- Angiotensin II inhibitors prevent angiotensin from attaching to the arteries.

Some Popular Blood Pressure Medications

- Diuretics: hydrochlorothiazide (Diuril)
- Beta-blockers: atenolol (Tenormin), propranolol hydrochloride (Inderal)

- Angiotensin converting enzyme (ACE) inhibitors: enalapril maleate (Vasotec), captopril (Capoten)
- Calcium channel blockers: diltiazem, hydrochloride (Cardizem CD)
- Vasodilators: hydralazine hydrochloride (Apresoline), minoxidil (Loniten)
- Central nervous system agents: alphamethyldopa (Aldomet)
- Angiotensin II inhibitors: valsartan (Diovan), losartan potassium (Cozaar)

Medication is an effective means of blood pressure control and management. However, there are several medications on the market, and research continually shows that these medications and their effects on blood pressure control vary from individual to individual.

For example, Ofili et al. (2013) stated that renin-angiotensin system (RAS) has been shown to be less effective in decreasing blood pressure in African Americans and obese people when it is given as monotherapy. But African Americans tend to react better to diuretics or calcium channel blockers (CCBs) than other classes of blood pressure medication. However, the authors stated that a thiazide-type diuretic along with a RAS inhibitor or CCB is an option that is often recommended for hypertension treatment. Ofili and colleagues pointed to the Anglo Scandinavian Cardiac Outcomes Trial that suggested that using "the RAS inhibitor as a second line agent may not be an optimal treatment approach in African Americans" (p. 3). It is the authors' belief that thiazide-type diuretics may be linked with adverse metabolic effects and may not be safe. This is especially so for obese people or those with dysglycemia, while RAS inhibitors use metabolic effects that are favorable and CCBs, for the most part, are considered metabolically neutral.

Ofili et al. (2013) conducted a post hoc analysis of the VITAE trial, a 16-week, double-blind, randomized forced-titration study. The study purpose was to determine whether the blood pressure-lowering effect of the combination of valsartan/hydrochlorothiazide was similar to amlodipine/hydrochlorothiazide for whites and African Americans who were not diabetic, but had hypertension and abdominal obesity. Subjects consisted of 126 African Americans and 212 whites. Subjects were 40 years old and older. There were more white males randomized to valsartan/hydrochlorothiazde in comparison to amlodipine/hydrochlorothiazide. The average baseline age of African American subjects was 53 years of age, 78 percent were women, most were obese with a mean body mass index (BMI) of 37 kg/m_2, and 63 percent had cardiometabolic syndrome. White subjects' average age was almost 58 years old, 61 percent were women, 75 percent had cardiometabolic syndrome and their average BMI was 35 kg/m_2.

Subjects received either combination therapy with valsartan/hydrochlorothiazide or monotherapy with hydrochlorothiazide from the beginning of the treatment to week eight. Then all subjects had combination therapy valsartan/hydrochlorothiazide or amlodipine/hydrochlorothiazide at week eight and ongoing. Subjects took their medication every day and at the same time every morning. Subjects had their blood pressure assessed both at baseline and then every four weeks afterwards. It is important to note that the arm that had the higher blood pressure reading when each subject was enrolled was used for all the following blood pressure measurements. Twenty-four-hour ambulatory blood pressure was also measured in a subset of subjects. To determine metabolic parameters, subjects had oral glucose tolerance tests done at baseline but at week 16 they fasted overnight for an assessment of fasting and postprandial glucose and insulin levels. It was important for the researchers to check and record adverse effects throughout the entire study. As a result, all observed or volunteered adverse events as well as serious AEs were documented. Also, physical examination was done at baseline, during the screening process and at various levels of the study.

Ofili et al. (2013) found that blood pressure-lowering effects were noted in prediabetic, obese hypertensive African Americans who had a combination of valsartan/hydrochlorothiazide, and the effects were similar to that of amlodipine/hydrochlorothiazide. It was shown that mean sitting systolic blood pressure and mean sitting diastolic blood pressure decreased with these treatment regimens. Blood pressure control was less than 140/90 mm Hg at the end of study. Further, both medication treatments had decreased both 24-hour ambulatory systolic blood pressure and diastolic blood pressure. Even though the blood pressure-lowering effects of both clinic and ambulatory valsartan/hydrochlorothiazide and amlodipine/hydrochlorothiazide were similar in African Americans, the efficiency of blood pressure-lowering was better for white subjects who had valsartan/hydrochlorothiazide than amlodipine/hydrochlorothiazide. When valsartan but not amlodipine was added to African American and white group treatment, valsartan reduced the hyperglycemic response to hydrochlorothiazide through enhanced secretion of insulin, reducing the negative metabolic effects linked with thiazide treatment. Similar observation was noted in both groups.

According to Wikoff et al. (2013), "metabolomics is a global biochemical approach that provides powerful tools for defining perturbations in metabolic pathways and networks in human disease" (p. 1).

In a similar racial and ethnic group metabolomics study regarding subjects' treatment response to antihypertensive medication, Wikoff et al. (2013) utilized a mass spectrometry-based metabolomics approach, considered a global biochemical approach. This was to explore biochemical changes in the metabolomics induced by a beta-adrenergic receptor called atenolol and to determine whether metabolomics gives insight about racial differences in drug response. The study was carried out on 272 Caucasians and African Americans with mild to moderate essential hypertension who participated in the Pharmacogenomic Evaluation of Antihypertensive Response study. There were 150 Caucasian subjects and 122 African American subjects. Plasma samples were collected and analyzed from subjects prior to and after the nine weeks of treatment with atenolol.

Wifkoff and colleagues found that both African American and Caucasian subjects' systolic and diastolic blood pressure was lowered, as well as subjects' LDL, HDL and plasma renin activity, while glucose, triglycerides and uric acid were higher during the nine weeks of the study period.

The differences in metabolic response of atenolol treatment in Caucasian and African American subjects were huge. The result showed a powerful effect of atenolol on fatty acids in Caucasian but not African American subjects. After subjects received atenolol treatment, free fatty acids, including saturated (palmitic), monounsaturated (oleic, palmitoleic) and polyunsaturated (arachidonic, linoleic), were lowered in Caucasians. But it was not so for African Americans. The effects of atenolol were either minimal or not present in this group. In a similar fashion, the study also demonstrated a significant 33 percent decrease of ketone body 3-hydroxybutyrate in whites. Again, this was not noted in African Americans. When the genetic variation in genes that encode lipases in Caucasians and African Americans was examined, the gene fragment SNP rs9652472 in LIPC was shown to be connected with oleic acid change only in Caucasian subjects. However, PLA2GC SNP rs7250148 was associated with oleic acid change in African American subjects.

The observed data signifies that atenolol-induced changes in the subjects' metabolome were race and genotype dependent. The authors stated that atenolol monotherapy is less effective to decrease blood pressure in people of African origin than in people of Caucasian descent. They believed that the differences in race in plasma renin activity are linked with the difference in response to antihypertensives. As a result, the authors concluded that there is a need to understand in detail the genetic or biochemical factors that support the differences in response.

JNC 8 Guidelines

Most practitioners today follow the JNC 8 guidelines when choosing appropriate hypertension medications for their patients. In their summary the JNC 8 Committee provided 9 graded recommendations on the basis of the strength of the available evidence used to make the recommendation: grade A indicates strong evidence, grade B moderate evidence, grade C weak evidence, and grade E of expert opinion in lieu of sufficient evidence.

Recommendation 1. Initiation of drug therapy to lower a systolic BP (SBP) of ≥150 mm Hg or a diastolic BP (DBP) of ≥ 90 mm Hg for the general population at 60 years of age or older (Grade A). A corollary recommendation is for patients already on pharmacological treatment who meet this goal to remain on current therapy if it is well tolerated.

Recommendation 2. For patients younger than 60 years, initiation of drug therapy when DBP is > 90 mm Hg. For patients between 18 and 29 years, the recommendation is based on expert opinion (Grade E).

Recommendation 3. For patients younger than 60 years, a SBP ≥140 mm Hg indicates therapy should be initiated.

Recommendation 4. In patients 18 years or older with chronic kidney disease (CKD), therapy should be used to lower a SBP >140 mm Hg with the goal of reducing SBP to < 140 mm Hg and DBP <90 mm Hg.

Recommendation 5. For the diabetic population ages 18 years and older, therapy should be instituted to lower blood pressure to < 140/90 mm Hg.

Recommendation 6. Initial drug therapy for nonblack patients (including those with diabetes) should include a thiazide-type diuretic, a CCB, an ACE inhibitor, or an ARB.

Recommendation 7. Initial drug therapy for black patients should include a thiazide-type diuretic or a CCB (Grade B with grade C for diabetic black patients).

Recommendation 8. For patients 18 years or older with CKD, initial or additional therapy should include an ACE inhibitor or ARB, regardless of race or diabetic status (Grade B).

Recommendation 9. An algorithm for managing patients who do not achieve control within one month of instituting therapy is recommended. This includes increasing the dose of the initial drug or adding a second drug from one of the other classes in recommendation 6. A third drug should be added if the goal is not achieved in one month using 2 drugs. Drugs from other classes can be used if drugs from the recommended drug classes are unsuccessful. Note that ACE inhibitors should not be combined with ARBs in the same patient. In complicated cases, a referral should be made to a hypertension specialist (Grade E). (Hernandez-Vila, 2015; James et al., 2015; Madhur and Maron 2014).

Resistant Hypertension

The literature also points to the potential benefit of treatment with the use of triple medications for people with resistant hypertension. "Among treated, uncontrolled hypertensive patients, the proportion on greater than three medications increased from 16 percent in 1988 to 1994 to 28 percent in 2005 to 2008" (Egan et al., 2013, p. 691). According to Azzi et al. (2014), surveys, tertiary centers and randomized trials showed that resistant hypertension prevalence ranges from 10 to 30 percent.

In a review of several large-scale population studies such as the US National Health and Nutrition Examination Survey (NHANES), researchers found the prevalence of resistant hypertension in adults with hypertension to be 8–12 percent. (Sarafidis et al., 2013). In this study researchers determined that the prevalence of resistant hypertension contrasts with the general improvement in blood pressure control rates during the same period (2010–2012). Sarafidis and his colleagues determined that the risk of cardiovascular events compared to nonresistant hypertensive patients is higher in patients older than 55 years and in patients of black ethnicity with high BMI, diabetes or chronic kidney disease. The investigators cautioned that data analyses that exclude the effects of white-coat hypertension and pseudoresistant hypertension are needed to clarify the epidemiology of true resistant hypertension.

In addition, for people with difficult-to-control blood pressure, the prevalence of end organ damage is greater. This is especially so for conditions such as left ventricular hypertrophy, and the incidence rate for cardiovascular events is greater when compared to patients with blood pressures that are better controlled.

Azzi et al. (2014) conducted a 12-week randomized, controlled, open, blinded endpoint trial study to compare the effects of two different treatment strategies in subjects with resistant hypertension. The treatment strategies were mineralocorticoid receptor blockade (MRB) and dual renin-angiotensin system blockade (RASB). The researchers wanted to compare their efficacy on blood pressure and the safety of the two strategies in subjects with resistance hypertension. The strategies utilized "the sequential use of aldosterone blockade and diuretic reinforcement or the sequential use of different renin-angiotensin system blockade" (p. 2039). Azizi et al. (2014) reported the effects of the utilized strategies on left ventricular (LV) mass in subjects with resistant hypertension. Subjects were 18 to 75 years old, male and female, resistant to three or more antihypertensive medications, including a diuretic, had supine office blood pressure of about 140 and/or 90 mm Hg and were referred to a tertiary care hypertension clinic. Subjects had both supine and 24-hour ambulatory blood pressure measured and monitored. Subjects were randomized to two groups, the MRB-based treatment group and RASB-based treatment group. It is important to note that some subjects had transthoracic echocardiography at baseline and at the 12-week follow-up visit.

Of the 167 subjects, baseline and echocardiographic examinations were made of 46 subjects in the MRB group and 40 subjects in the RASB group. But there was no significant difference in baseline clinical characteristics and laboratory parameters between these 86 subjects and those 81 subjects who had no baseline and final echocardiographic examinations. It was also shown that there was not a significant difference in baseline echocardiographic parameters between both groups.

The addition of spironolactone at a low dosage to triple treatment therapy that includes an ARB, then by progressive titrated sodium reduction, demonstrated a larger decrease in ambulatory blood pressure than increasing RASB with an additional ACE inhibitor and a beta-blocker. LV mass index reduction with MRB was assisted by lower LV filling. Interestingly, it was revealed that the greater improvement of echocardiographic parameters with MRB rather than RASB was related to the huge decrease in blood pressure that was obtained with MRB.

Azzi et al. (2014) believed that the difference in LV mass index reduction between MRB and RASB treatment groups remains significant even after adjustment for low blood pressure. They suggested that there is "a direct myocardial structural effect on MR blockade per se, because of neutralization of the direct effects of aldosterone (or other steroids) on the heart, including inflammation, fibrosis and hypertrophy" (p. 2042). These effects may have played a role in the effective benefits of MRB in relation to decreasing cardiovascular illnesses and death. The authors pointed to the result that showed MRB treatment having quick effects on LV mass index during subjects' 12-week study treatment.

The researchers concluded that a strategy that is based on MRB and diuretic treatment quickly lowers LV mass index more effectively than a strategy that is based on maximum RASB in subjects with resistance hypertension. Additionally, the findings give an extra reason for prescribing MRBs for people with resistance hypertension.

It is reported by Egan et al. (2013) that "30 to 50 percent of patients with treatment-resistant hypertension (TRH) are pseudoresistant, i.e., nonadherent and/or out-of-office blood pressure nonhypertensive" (p. 691). The percentage of TRH patients on suboptimal treatment regimens is unknown, as are the clinical characteristics of these individuals and the clinical factors that correspond with optimal therapy in the primary care settings. They believed that if these factors are recognized, the data could help with the development of strategies to improve hypertension control in the broad cluster of people with uncontrolled hypertension, in particular people on suboptimal regimens.

Egan et al. (2013) utilized electronic data from 468,877 subjects at 200 clinical sites in the Outpatient Quality Improvement Network from 2007 to 2010. Subjects were age 18 years or older and diagnosed with hypertension. The purpose was to explain the percentage of uncontrolled hypertensive subjects with apparent TRH on prescribed optimal regimens, and also to establish the clinical factors that were independently associated with optimal therapy.

It is important to note that the authors used apparent TRH only because treatment adherence as well as measurement artifacts were not available in the electronic data from their study sites. Also, blood pressure control was defined as blood pressure of less than 140/90 mm Hg for this study.

The study showed that in the community-based practice network of the controlled and uncontrolled hypertensive subjects grouped by the amount of antihypertensive medication they were prescribed, hypertensive subjects whose blood pressure was controlled were prescribed fewer antihypertensive drugs. However, they were more likely to be taking a statin cholesterol-lowering medication. Nevertheless, it was revealed that apparent TRH was prevalent in the group with uncontrolled hypertension. The reason was related to the 468,877 subjects with hypertension. It was shown that 31.5 percent (147,635 subjects) had blood pressure that was uncontrolled. Among subjects with uncontrolled blood pressure, 30.3 percent (44,684) were prescribed three or more blood pressure medications. Of these, only 22,189 subjects (15.0 percent) were prescribed an optimal regimen.

In terms of clinical factors that were independently linked with prescribed optimal blood pressure therapy, it was demonstrated that higher CVD and CHD risk, black race, diabetes mellitus and CKD were associated factors in hypertensive subjects. Of interest, for black subjects with both controlled and uncontrolled apparent TRH, blood pressure was less likely to be controlled compared to their white counterparts; however, they were more likely to be prescribed an optimal therapy.

In this study, the clinical factors that were most and strongly independently connected with blood pressure control in subjects with apparent TRH were CVD and a prescribed single pill of combined antihypertensive medication and statins. According to the authors, their article confirmed prior reports that showed that the use of single-pill combinations and the prescription of statins among white people were associated with improved blood pressure control.

The authors stated that for subjects with uncontrolled blood pressure on optimal therapy, "strategies to select more efficacious regimens represent a potentially effective option" (Egan et al., 2013, p. 696). They also believed that other factors that may have controlled blood pressure in subjects with apparent TRH involved the controlled subset. For example, the controlled subset subjects were likely to have aldosterone antagonists and loop diuretics compared to uncontrolled subjects, but controlled subjects were not more likely to get thiazide diuretics compared to uncontrolled apparent TRH subjects. Common medications prescribed in both controlled and uncontrolled apparent TRH subjects were diuretics, ACE inhibitors, calcium channel blockers, beta-blockers and angiotensin receptor blockers.

In this study there was a low proportion of apparent TRH subjects who were prescribed aldosterone antagonists. This led Egan et al. (2013) to conclude that aldosterone antagonists could be beneficial for a larger proportion of subjects, given that both aldosterone antagonists and loop diuretics are powerful strategies for people with apparent TRH. The recent guidelines and statements recommend a renin-angiotensin system blocker, calcium channel blocker and a diuretic in a triple drug regimen.

In a similar study, Kent et al. (2014) looked at the classes of antihypertensive medication filled among U.S. Medicare beneficiaries who were initiating treatment. They also evaluated the association between subjects' demographics and comorbidities with the initiation of antihypertensive medication classes. The researchers analyzed a 5 percent random sample of Medicare beneficiaries from the Centers for Medicare and Medicaid Services. Subjects were age 65 or older, had initiated antihypertensive medication between 2007 and 2010, had two or more outpatient visits with a diagnosis of hypertension, and had full Medicare fee-for-service coverage for the 365 days before they initiated antihypertensive medication.

For this study, the definition of initiation was the first antihypertensive medication fill followed by 365 days with no medication being filled. Results showed that 32,142 (61.9 percent) subjects began taking antihypertensive medications. However, in 2010, of subjects who had initiated antihypertensive medications, 31.3 percent filled prescription for ACE inhibitors (ACE-1), 26.9 percent filled beta-blockers, 17.2 percent calcium channel blockers, while 14.4 percent had filled angiotensin receptor blockers (ARBs). Older subjects were less likely to initiate an ACE-1 or thiazide-type diuretic for their treatment. When comparing black and white subjects, it was less likely for black subjects to initiate an ACE-1 or loop diuretic for their treatment. However, thiazide-type diuretics or calcium channel blockers (CCB) were more likely to be initiated by black subjects.

When whites were compared with Hispanic subjects, Hispanics were more likely to initiate ACE-1 or ARB medication classes, but less likely to initiate a loop or potassium-sparing diuretic. Asian subjects were more likely to initiate an ARB or CCB medication than whites, but least likely to initiate an ACE-1 loop diuretic for their treatment.

It was also shown that those beneficiaries with a Medicaid buy-in were least likely to initiate an ARB or thiazide-type or potassium-spring diuretic; rather the likelihood was greater that they would use a loop diuretic for initiation of therapy.

Subjects with diabetes were more likely to initiate an ACE-1 for therapy but were least likely to initiate therapy with a thiazide-type or CCB when compared to those who were not diabetic. Similarly, subjects with conditions such as CHD, stroke, CKD or heart failure were least likely to initiate their treatment with an ARB or a thiazide-type diuretic than those without these conditions. However, those with these conditions were more likely to initiate therapy with loop diuretic or beta-blocker classes of drug.

Nonetheless, when comparing black subjects to white subjects, the overall finding was that initiation of more than one antihypertensive medication class was reduced from 2007 to 2010. For example, it decreased from 25 percent in 2007 to 24.1 percent in 2010. Subjects had initiated more than one antihypertensive medication for therapy and of these, the most prevalent class was a thiazide-type diuretic and either an ACE-1 or ARB class of antihypertensive medication.

The authors also found that thiazide-type diuretic initiation was slightly decreased between 2007 and 2010, and the information obtained from their study showed that 31 percent and 17 percent of subjects, respectively, had initiated an ACE-1 or CCB for antihypertensive treatment. Subjects who had initiated antihypertensive medication initiated a class of antihypertensive drugs that had been recommended by the Eighth Joint National Committee (JNC 8). But 30 percent had initiated antihypertensive medication with the use of drug classes that have not been recommended by the JNC 8. The Seventh Report of the Joint National Committee on the Prevention, Detection, Evaluation, and Treatment of High Blood Pressure (JNC 7) guidelines for the prevention and treatment of hypertension had recommended a thiazide-type diuretic. The guideline indicates that this should be given to people who are newly diagnosed with hypertension as the first-line therapy, whereas the present JNC 8 guidelines indicate that people who are not black, and diabetics should include a thiazide-type diuretic, CCB, ACE-1 or ARB drug classes.

According to Kent et al. (2014), the initial antihypertensive treatment should include a thiazide-type diuretic or CCB for black people. It was shown that 34.3 percent of the subjects with CKD had initiated antihypertensive medications that utilized an ACE-1 or ARB treatment therapy (30.7 percent in blacks, 34.9 percent in nonblacks with CKD). Importantly, these drug classes had been recommended by the JNC 8.

A Glance: Hypertension Management by Various Hypertension Societies

Different agencies in both affluent and less affluent countries across the globe have published hypertension management guidelines. These guidelines are written by expert groups established by national and regional authorities (Chalmers, Arima, Harrap, Touyz & Park, 2013). For instance, committees that establish management guidelines can be assigned by either health authorities or professional medical groups such as Societies of Hypertension. These guidelines are generally updated every 3 to 5 years (Chalmers et al., 2013). Despite the updated guidelines, Chalmers et al. (2013) stated that they are not necessarily current, based on the most recent research from "large-scale randomized trials, observational studies or meta-analyses" (p. 1043).

According to the authors, the Forum of the International Society of Hypertension (ISH) put together experts from different hypertension agencies connected to ISH. At present, there are 90 professional expert groups from 77 countries represented by a variety of different socioeconomic regions.

To determine the trends in documentation of changes in clinical practice for hypertension management, Chalmers et al. (2013) conducted a cross-sectional survey of national and regional societies affiliated with the ISH. Chalmers et al. (2013) utilized a formal questionnaire to carry out the survey in December 2011; 84 national and six regional societies from 77 countries were invited. The survey sought to find out present use of national, regional and international guidelines, the present use of blood pressure measurement, and the present recommendations on lifestyle measures, the preferred blood pressure-lowering drugs, and blood pressure thresholds and targets.

Thirty-one societies responded. Nine societies were from high-income countries, 17 from upper to middle-income countries, and five were from lower-middle or low-income countries, as defined by the World Bank.

Of the 31 societies, 21 societies used national guidelines, three used regional guidelines, and 17 used either international guidelines alone or supplementary guidelines.

In terms of current practices for blood pressure measurement, two-thirds utilized mercury, aneroid and semiautomatic sphygmomanometers, and half utilized ambulatory blood pressure monitoring (ABPM).

The study also revealed that all the nations had recommended lifestyle measures for hypertension management, but three nations (the Vietnamese Society of Hypertension, Taiwan Hypertension Society, and Swiss Society of Hypertension) had recommended lifestyle measures such as exercise, restriction of salt, and weight loss. But other measures, such as dietary programs, not smoking, moderate alcohol consumption and the control of stress, were used the least.

Almost all of the societies had reported extensive use of the drug classes. These drug classes were ACE inhibitors, ARBs, CCBs and diuretics. However, 12 societies out of 31 had not recommended beta-blockers. It is important to note that the use of CCBs and diuretics were largely used in elderly people, but the use of beta-blockers was not used in these individuals. Most importantly, it was reported that beta-blockers were recommended globally for people with CHD. It should be noted that beta blockers are no longer recommended as a first line of therapy for the management of hypertension in the United States (De Caterina and Leone 2010).

ACE inhibitors and ARBs were the preferred drugs used for people with conditions such as diabetes, renal disease, and metabolic syndrome. Surprisingly, most nations' favorite was combination therapy of RAS inhibitors with either CCBs or diuretics, whereas a solid majority had reported a preference of combined CCB with RAS inhibitors for people with type 2 diabetes.

In terms of threshold for initiating hypertension drug therapy, blood pressure of 140/90 mm Hg was used by most societies for people without complications. However, half had retained the previous threshold of 130/80 mm Hg for initiating drug treatment in people who were considered high risk. These were individuals with conditions such as CHD, stroke or type 2 diabetes.

The differences in treatment across countries as well as countries with varying income levels were consistent, with the exception of ABPM and moderation of alcohol consumption recommendations. These two measures were least prevalent in areas with fewer resources and usage of CCB for obese people, yet these were not so common in the wealthier nations.

Chalmers et al. (2013) emphasized the need for basic guidelines that would fit well in low-income areas worldwide. Further, attention should be focused on those countries that do not have resources to build their own national recommendations.

Differences in Medication Response in Non-Hispanic Whites and African Americans

Researchers continue to document various reasons why some people with hypertension respond better to some blood pressure medications. Canzanello et al. (2008) believed that if the clinical factors that are linked to how blood pressure reacts to each drug class are established, control rates could be increased. Also, there could be improvement on the present "trial and error" method of choosing drug therapy for people with hypertension, Canzanello et al. (2008) studied women and men between the ages of 30 and 59. Participants consisted of African Americans and non-Hispanic whites. The purpose was to study the characteristics that may be predictive factors of blood pressure response in both groups who had essential hypertension and were treated with candesartan medication (32 mg daily) for a six-week period after participants had a drug-free washout period of at least four weeks (baseline). Measurements at enrollment, baseline, and end of treatment were covered to determine the predictive response for this study.

The study revealed that non Hispanic ethnicity and higher seated plasma renin activity (PRA) values were shown to be predictive of a greater response to the renin-angiotensin-aldosterone system (RAAS) antagonist drug candesartan. For instance, in non-Hispanic white women, the systolic blood pressure decrease was greater compared to non-Hispanic white men and African American men and women. Also, in non-Hispanic white women, diastolic blood pressure was greatly reduced compared to African American men and women. But the diastolic decrease in non-Hispanic white women was not more than in non-Hispanic white men. It was also shown that there was significantly higher blood pressure in non-Hispanic white men than in male and female African American participants.

According to Canzanello et al. (2008), their findings show that "easily obtained demographics, clinical and laboratory" data can provide significant observation of blood pressure response to candesartan treatment in people with essential hypertension. They further reported that a combination of all predictors such as ethnicity, gender, ethnicity-gender interaction, weight, baseline blood pressure, seated PRA, and the change in PRA in response to candesartan accounted for 39 percent of the individual variation in both systolic and diastolic blood pressure responses.

Medication Adherence

A body of literature has outlined several factors regarding adherence to medication regimes for effective blood pressure control and management.

Many of these factors are complex. But it is important to establish why some people adhere and why others do not. Having an understanding of these factors and patients' perceptions of their health condition could increase awareness. Similarly, the implementation of community measures could also be an effective tool to assist people to cope and manage their chronic illness. If the whys behind adherence are fully understood, health care providers involved in patient care together with the patient could increase adherence. For instance, studies show "that patients tend to adhere better the closer they are to visiting their doctor" (Stavropoulou, 2011, p. 189). As a result, surveys that are done in a clinical setting just before or after people have had a consultation visit yield greater reported adherence rates (Stavropoulou, 2011).

According to Park et al. (2014) adherence is "the extent to which a person's behavior, such as taking medicine, corresponds with the agreed recommendations of a health care provider, implicating the active involvement of patients in medication-taking behavior" (p. 18).

Stringent adherence to medication regimen is of utmost importance for blood pressure control. While some people may find taking antihypertensive medications on a daily basis an obstacle, the long-term effects of hypertension risk can be more difficult. The two serious complications of uncontrolled hypertension are stroke and cardiovascular diseases (Stavropoulou, 2011).

A blister pack would be a very useful tool to help with organizing medications. A local drugstore pharmacist can assist people to prepare medications in a blister pack and will most likely answer their questions related to medications. This well-known medication tool can be purchased at a drugstore pharmacy. The most people can do is ask questions, especially if they are struggling with organizing and remembering their blood pressure medications. An illustration of a blister pack is shown in figure 10.

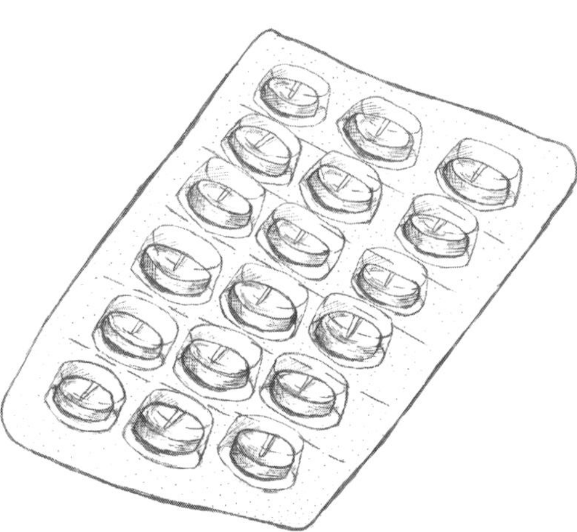

Figure 10. A blister pack is used for organizing and managing medications. This tool helps people organize their medications and remember to take them, especially if they take a lot. Medication is accessed by pushing through the foil (courtesy Dominique Diedrick).

The study by Park et al. (2014) was conducted in Seoul on older Korean adults 65 years and older with hypertension. This study looked at factors that contributed to antihypertensive medication adherence. The authors examined whether socioeconomic characteristics, disease-related characteristics, knowledge, antihypertensive lifestyle, and memory contributed significantly to medication adherence among these participants.

Park et al. (2014) demonstrated that of the two groups, the adherent and nonadherent groups, no difference in knowledge was observed. In terms of lifestyle, individuals in the adherent group had a shorter time since they were diagnosed and a shorter time span of using antihypertensive medication. Not only were these similarities noted in this group of participants, but their systolic and diastolic blood pressures were reduced compared to the nonadherent group.

Participants in the adherent group had a higher total metamemory score as shown on the perception of memory ability scale. Univariate analysis demonstrated that better memory function was an important predictor of better antihypertensive medication adherence. Overall, the adherence rate with antihypertensive medication was 59 percent and 41 percent nonadherent. Seventy-five percent of participants were 75 years or older, while 60 percent were males. Multiple factors were related to adherence to antihypertensive medication in the univariate and multivariate analysis. These were employment status, individuals' adherence to an antihypertensive lifestyle, and metamemory.

The participants that had practiced antihypertensive health behaviors were more likely to adhere to antihypertensive medication. Lifestyle behaviors participants had pursued were low-sodium diet, regular exercise, and going for regular clinic visits. It was interesting to note that this study showed that adult participants who were older and were employed were more likely to be adherent compared to unemployed adult participants.

The authors emphasized the need to continue supporting older people with this condition to increase blood pressure control and to attain long-term adherence.

When it comes to chronic illnesses, adherence treatment consists of a protocol involving several measures, for example, diet, exercise and medication (Pasucci et al., 2010). It is also believed by these authors that nonadherence to drug therapy has been constantly associated with taking a lot of medication and the complexity of the medication regimen. But other studies have pointed to other reasons for patient nonadherence to medication.

Factors or Barriers to Medication Adherence for Hypertension in Different Cultural Groups

Lewis, Askie, Randleman and Shelton-Dunston (2010) showed that hypertensive African Americans had reported a number of contextual factors that were described as most salient barriers to medication adherence. First, limited financial resources were a factor for nonadherence. But it was mostly due to the stress they perceived that comes with the decision regarding where to put their limited resources and not the funds to purchase their medication. As a result, subjects saw this as a barrier that reduced their desire to stay adherent. It has been reported that in the general population, an estimated 40 percent of nonadherence is due to inability to afford medications (Cuffee et al., 2013). Other barriers according to Lewis et al. (2010) were neighborhood violence and distrust of healthcare providers.

Similar studies on African Americans regarding antihypertension adherence have been reported. For example, Gross et al. (2103) stated that barriers such as real or imagined side effects and the preference of home remedies instead of prescribed medications were reasons for nonadherence. Further, Leung et al. (2012) have listed several reasons for medication nonadherence in patients with hypertension.

According to Leung et al. (2012), these are "financial cost of medication, long duration of drug therapy, lack of symptoms in hypertension, complicated drug regimens, not understanding hypertension management, lack of motivation, and conflicting individual health beliefs" (Leung et al., 2012, p. 20).

Although it is vital for people to adhere to treatment measures to maintain effective blood pressure levels, of nonadherence to antihypertensive medication is prevalent in some countries such as the United States and Taiwan (Li et al., 2012). Even though a range of antihypertensive medications exist to treat people with hypertension and these antihypertensive medications are reported to be effective, about one-third of Taiwanese are adherent to taking their medication for blood pressure control (Li et al., 2012). Wikoff et al. (2013) also reported that despite the availability of many antihypertensive drug classes to treat hypertension, only approximately 50 percent of patients experience decreased blood pressure with any of the medication provided for treatment, and less than 40 percent of people with this condition have controlled blood pressure.

A study was conducted by Holt et al. (2013) on adult men and women age 65 and older who were being treated for essential hypertension. The purpose of the study was to determine whether factors such as sociodemographics (e.g., age, race, marital status, education, height and weight to calculate BMI, clinical, health care system, psychosocial, and behavioral factors) were differentially associated with low antihypertensive medication adherence scores. Holt et al. (2013) defined low antihypertensive medication adherence as a score less than six based on the eight-item Morisky Medication Adherence Scale (MMAS-8); data were gathered about risk factors of low adherence by telephone surveys and administrative databases.

Holt et al. (2013) found that factors that were associated with low adherence scores in men were prescription cost and lower sexual functioning, which men found to be a barrier to antihypertensive adherence. Men with higher BMI also had lower medication adherence. The findings also showed that depressive symptoms in women were associated with low adherence, and the cost of antihypertensive medications was also a factor. Importantly, women, but not men, reported that they were dissatisfied with communication with their health care providers and this was a barrier to adherence. In addition, both male and female participants who practiced fewer lifestyle modifications to control their blood pressure tended to have low adherence scores.

Holt et al. (2013) concluded that if providers explained the importance of medication adherence, especially when women are assessed at clinic visits, the interaction would probably enhance adherence and control of blood pressure. Similarly, providers should engage in discussions with patients to identify adherence issues related to cost. The researchers also reported that "identifying and addressing any perceived sexual side effects for antihypertensive medications might successfully improve adherence behavior in men" (p. 562).

A similar study was conducted by Li et al. (2012) on 200 Taiwanese hypertensive participants 18 years and older. Participants were recruited from a large teaching hospital in northern Taiwan. This study utilized self-administered questionnaires, review of participants' medical charts and blood pressure measurements taken twice for each participant. The researchers examined the prevalence of antihypertensive medication nonadherence and how the cultural/clinical factors were associated with nonadherence in Taiwan.

The findings of the study indicated two factors that were associated with medication nonadherence in this group. It was found that participants who had perceived lower susceptibility to complications from having hypertension had the worse medication adherence. Secondly, those who had a hypertension diagnosis for a longer length of time were the least adherent to taking Western antihypertensive medications. It was revealed that out of the 200 participants, only 49 percent, which was considered low, had their blood pressure controlled, and medication adherence was shown in 47.5 percent of participants. This was also considered a low percentage.

It was noted that health-related social support and social support in general had no significant association with medication adherence. This study looked at two social support measures, for example, support provided not only by family members but also relatives and friends. The majority of the study participants were married (86 percent) or lived with families (94 percent).

The researchers stated that their results could be of importance for other researchers and clinicians in terms of providing intervention. The intervention can enable patients to enhance their management of hypertension by including family members in their care, as demonstrated in the Western population, but not in the Taiwanese group. For instance, in China only 17.0 percent of participants used Chinese herbs to promote their health or treat their disease (e.g., cough) in combination with their antihypertensive medications. Because of this low percentage of participants that used Chinese herbs in this study compared to Chinese herb usage of Chinese immigrants in the United States (43 percent), Li et al. (2012) stated that the Taiwanese may not perceive much benefit in using Chinese herbs compared to Chinese immigrants living in the United States. The researchers emphasized that it should not be assumed by clinicians and researchers that these groups perceive health care the same way, even though Taiwanese people may share similar Chinese cultural values with immigrant Chinese residing in the United States.

This study provides relevant cultural information, which can educate healthcare providers who treat people of different cultural backgrounds. The study results should not be limited to people of Taiwanese descent because other groups may have similar experiences or views about hypertension. This study suggests that the implementation of knowledge should be broad, because patient care is provided at different spectrums in the health care environment, such as hospitals, clinics, and communities. If healthcare workers acquire a better insight into people's health concerns and their perception of health, they may be able to facilitate increased awareness.

In the same manner, educating patients about the potential complications of uncontrolled or untreated hypertension and implementing strategies for effective blood pressure control could increase medication adherence in people with hypertension. Additionally, another good strategy is to introduce culturally sensitive care in nursing school curricula since nurses play a crucial role in the care of people with various health conditions, including hypertension.

Stavropoulou (2011) studied patients in Athens, Greece, in the Center for the Treatment of Hypertension at Hippokration General Hospital. The researcher examined subjects' perception regarding differences between information needs for hypertension and medication to treat it as well as the resources subjects used to obtain information about hypertension, and they explored whether it was information about hypertension or the medication that was more important to them in determining nonadherence to their prescribed antihypertensive medication.

Stavropoulou (2011) utilized the Morisky scale to measure nonadherence in subjects. This scale consisted of four yes or no questions about medication usage. Stavropoulou found that of the 743 subjects that participated in the study, 90 percent reported that they felt well informed about hypertension, whereas 80 percent felt informed about medications they received to treat hypertension. It was interesting to note that subjects felt that they were better informed regarding hypertension compared to the medication that was used to treat their condition.

Regarding sources to acquire information about hypertension and medication to treat hypertension, subjects reported that the doctor was their main source of information.

The findings also showed that of the source choices (e.g., family/friends, doctor, pharmacist, nurse, other patients with hypertension, media such as television, radio and newspaper, and Internet, and magazines about health issues and nutrition), the media, including magazines on health issues and nutrition, were the second most often used source of information for hypertension reported by subjects. However, the sources of information pertaining to medication were few compared to sources for hypertension.

The researchers found that subjects who felt that they were well informed about medication for treating their condition were least nonadherent, while information about hypertension was not a predictor for nonadherence among subjects. The result of the study demonstrated that nonadherence was not a factor because subjects were mostly adherent.

This study suggests that socioeconomic status and subjects' cultural beliefs may have played a role in their perception of adherence. This may be due to the older age group (average age of 61) in this study, the high percentage of married subjects, and their level of education.

Compared to other studies that showed the opposite result to Stavropoulou's study, Lewis et al. (2010) stated that beliefs regarding hypertension and the medication for treating it influence how people manage their condition and adhere to the recommended treatment. These factors, they believed, are considered determinants of medication adherence. This study result showed several differences compared to Stavropoulou's study. For instance, most subjects reported mistrust of health care professionals in terms of what they had "perceived as racism and discrimination on the part of their doctor" (Lewis et al., 2010, p. 203). In Lewis et al. (2010), subjects were younger, mostly female, and had low income, while Stavropoulou's (2011) subjects were 40 percent male, the majority of subjects were married, and approximately half of the subjects felt they were able to cope with the current income in the home.

Factors that Affect Medication Adherence in African Americans with Hypertension

Schoenthaler et al. (2009) evaluated patients' perceptions of their providers' communication about medication adherence in African Americans who were 18 years and older, diagnosed with hypertension, and enrolled in a community-based health care practice in the New York metropolitan area. The study was carried out as part of an ongoing randomized, controlled trial, Counseling African Americans to Control Hypertension, based in Community/ Migrant Health Centers. African American subjects utilized a self-reported adherence questionnaire to report medication adherence. The Morisky Medication Adherence Scale measured adherence using a questionnaire that consisted of four "yes or no" response questions. These were (a) "Have you ever forgotten to take your blood pressure medicine?" (b) "Are you sometimes careless in regards to your medicine?" (c) "Do you skip your medicine when you are feeling well?" and (d) "When you feel badly due to the medicine, do you skip it?" The scale coded "1" for each negative response, thus a higher total score showed better adherence. Total scores ranged from 0 to 4. Subjects' ratings of their providers' communication was assessed with a perceived communication style questionnaire—a measure adapted from a study which assessed "the effect of physicians' initial and follow-up communication styles on the beliefs and behaviors of patients with depression" (Schoenthaler et al., 2009, p. 186).

Of interest, 72 providers were included in this study, and data from 439 subjects with poorly controlled hypertension was obtained and analyzed. Most providers were female and their average age was 45 years, whereas 68 percent of African American subjects were female and their average age was 58 years.

In terms of subjects' provider ratings, the study findings showed that provider communication that was perceived as more collaborative was significantly associated with better adherence to prescribed antihypertensive medications. It was also shown that younger subjects and those with depressive symptoms related better to the providers. It was noted that 55 percent of subjects reported they were nonadherent with their medications, whereas 51 percent had rated their providers' communication as noncollaborative. The authors stated that their additional study that adjusted for covariates, for example, depressive symptoms and medical comorbidity, may assist in the explanation of underlying mechanisms between patient-provider communication and medication adherence. The researchers concluded that it is vital to take into account the patient's perspective of the relationship between the patient and the provider (Schoenthaler et al., 2009, p. 18).

It is believed that when people with hypertension experience discrimination, the psychological response of the experience may have an impact on medication adherence. For example, Cuffee et al. (2013) examined whether reported racial discrimination was associated with medication nonadherence among 730 primary care African Americans with a mean age of 53 years.

Subjects were diagnosed with hypertension and were receiving care in an inner-city safety net setting. The researchers also sought to determine whether distrust of physicians was a contributing factor among this low-income group recruited in Birmingham, Alabama.

Cuffee et al. (2013) found that racial discrimination was associated with subjects' lower medication adherence. For instance, of the 730 subjects, 112 had reported low adherence to medication, 350 were nonadherent, and 318 were in adherence. Higher subject age, being male, and their trust with their physician were associated with increased adherence. It was also shown that general trust in physicians was associated with subjects' reported discrimination and medication adherence. In African American women, adherence rates were lower. Cuffee et al. (2013) believe that interventions to improve medication adherence could be strengthened by including trust-building components. In the same manner, if focus is directed to developing a patient-physician relationship that is culturally competent, this strategy probably will increase adherence in African American people. Cuffee et al. (2013) also believe that strategies to promote "earned trust" could also be beneficial for African American men and women.

Another study done by Manze, Rose, Orner, Berlowitz and Kressin (2010) explored the extent of racial disparities in treatment intensification (TI) in blood pressure control among 819 black and white participants. Subjects were 21 years and older, diagnosed with hypertension, and visited a primary care clinic at an urban safety net hospital.

Their findings demonstrated that those participants with concerns about their blood pressure medications and those with more provider counseling were both associated with lower TI. Black participants had more concerns about their medication, but their TI was lower than white participants, which was equivalent to almost one less therapy increase per 17 visits to the clinic. These participants also perceived that their blood pressure was more serious. Importantly, the result showed that blacks' systolic blood pressure was higher (134 mm Hg, compared to their white counterparts' average of 131 mm Hg). It was noted that blacks' adherence was more likely to be fair or poor, and they were least likely to have excellent adherence.

Differences between black and white participants regarding their hypertension-related beliefs were also found. Although all participants had agreed that their providers had understood their background and values, black participants agreed less strongly. Similarly, all participants disagreed that their provider looked down on them and the way they had lived their lives. But white participants more strongly disagreed. Belief examples reported by black participants in terms of the cause of their hypertension were germs or virus, chance, other people, and the medical care they had received in the past.

While more black participants reported that if they took their blood pressure medications they would feel better, they did not believe that the medications would help them to live a longer life.

It is important to note that one of the determinants for TI was hyperlipidemia. This condition was the only predictor.

The researchers stated that their findings add to the literature that shows determinants for TI by race and shows that participants' concerns and beliefs about blood pressure and provider counseling are linked with the different rates of TI. However, they emphasized that the findings should not be generalized to other populations, because only two groups were studied at a single location.

The finding suggested the need for more education and awareness at the provider's level if blood pressure is to be adequately controlled. If providers gain more understanding of black cultural beliefs about taking medication for blood pressure treatment, they may be better equipped to address their needs. Hopefully, the insight may help to decrease disparities in this unfortunate group with hypertension, given the ultimate goal is to control blood pressure and blood pressure-related complications.

In conclusion, black people need to be educated about hypertension, and they should understand that it is a serious chronic condition. Education should be focused on the importance of taking prescribed medication for blood pressure control, and such treatment should not be taken lightly. While it may be difficult to change medication beliefs, it is likely that some people may understand the significance of taking prescribed medication if a simple explanation is provided.

Elder et al. (2012) conducted a study on 235 Southern hypertensive African American men 18 years and older. Subjects were recruited from a safety net hospital in Birmingham, Alabama, from 2007 to 2010. The study assessed the relationship between trust in medical professionals, medication adherence and hypertension control among subjects.

The study revealed that subjects whose general trust in the medical system was higher had better medication adherence in comparison to those with lower trust. However, hypertension control had no association with the medical system. But, those with high self-efficacy were more likely to have better hypertension control when compared to subjects with lower self-efficacy. Subjects with higher self-efficacy were also more likely to have better medication adherence. Elder et al. (2012) concluded that there are no prior studies that "examined the relationship between trust, medication adherence, and hypertension control in African American men" (p. 2244). They believed that changes at the developmental stage of the health systems should be taken into consideration to foster trust in African American men when interventions are being developed to promote medication adherence.

9

Hypertension Case Stories

The Story of an African American Woman

When my family doctor told me that I had high blood pressure, I was not surprised but I felt really sad. Sometimes I had my blood pressure checked at my doctor's office or at a blood pressure stand in a health store or pharmacy department even before I was diagnosed. I always do some form of exercise like walking or running, and I take the stairs as often as I can.

My family doctor had informed me that my blood pressure was high on several occasions, and he had based it on what was considered the normal blood pressure value. However, he said that if I lost weight, cut back on salty foods, and exercised regularly, these things might help my blood pressure return to normal. He also said he would not have to prescribe medication to stabilize my blood pressure if it was within the normal range at the next follow-up visit. He strongly suggested I follow his recommendations.

I followed my doctor's advice. I tried a combination of natural home remedies that elderly folks in my culture use for high blood pressure, so that my blood pressure would be normal again and I would not have to take blood pressure pills. I lost some weight but not a significant amount. I continued to exercise and reduced the amount of salt in my diet.

When checked, my blood pressure would sometimes be within a normal range but at other times it was above normal readings. I had chest pain once and felt scared, so I went to my doctor for a checkup. He referred me to a cardiologist. The cardiologist asked me about my blood pressure measurement history, and I informed him that sometimes it was normal but that other times it was not.

I was not that surprised when I was diagnosed with hypertension, because I had several close family members with high blood pressure and some were diagnosed at an earlier age than I had been. I thought it would be difficult to remember to take blood pressure pills every day, and I don't like taking pills.

So, I thought if I were more serious about changing my diet and losing more weight, my blood pressure might level off within an acceptable range.

The cardiologist sent his report to my family doctor and told me he would suggest that my family doctor start me on a mild, low-dose diuretic to keep my pressure within normal range. He said that it would help to preserve my kidneys. I went for a follow-up with my family doctor and he said the test I had had at the cardiologist's was normal. He then checked my blood pressure and again it was not within normal range. I told him what the cardiologist suggested, and he read the cardiologist's report.

My family doctor told me that I had high blood pressure, and he started me on a blood pressure medication called hydrochlorothiazide, which I took every day. I felt sad that I had to take a pill every day, but if my blood pressure is controlled, I can still live a normal life. Also, I may not end up having a stroke or developing kidney problems.

I have accepted that I have high blood pressure. I also realize that it is chronic; therefore, I have no choice but to take my medication exactly as my doctor prescribed. I also modified my diet to include more fruits and vegetables. I eat more high-fiber, low-fat foods and have cut down on salt in my diet. I exercise by running on my treadmill one to two times every week for 30 to 35 minutes each time. I also jog in the summer one or two times a week for at least 30 to37 minutes each time, and I am still trying to lose more weight.

I am taking two different types of blood pressure pills now. In addition to watching what I eat, I continue to monitor my blood pressure at home, at the doctor's office and at a pharmacy. I put my blood pressure medication bottles on my kitchen counter every night so I can see them in the morning when I go into the kitchen to prepare my breakfast. Once I take my pills, I put the bottles back in the cupboard. This prevents me from missing a day of medication. Sometimes you have to help yourself when you have a serious health problem like high blood pressure.

The Case of Jasper (J.M.)

J.M. is a 68-year-old retired African American male. He has kidney disease, hypertension and insulin-dependent diabetes. He has no vision in his left eye and only 40 percent vision in the right eye. His medications are Humalog (insulin) twice a day, Coversyl, and calcium pills. He used to take baby aspirin every day, but he recently stopped. He said the aspirin tablet was to prevent a heart attack, because he is at a greater risk for heart disease.

J.M. developed kidney disease in 2001, and at this time his kidneys had started to fail. They finally failed fully on April 4, 2011, three years after he had developed diabetes. He developed diabetes, then hypertension. He had a cough that he thought was a cold, but his doctor told him that it was water around his lungs. His other symptoms were general weakness and the sensation of a lot of fluid inside his body. His family doctor referred him to a hospital, and then the hospital specialist referred him to a renal clinic.

He began going to a renal clinic in 2001 and was started on hemodialysis treatment in April of 2011, when his kidneys failed. When he was told that his kidneys had failed at the renal clinic, J.M. said he was devastated.

J.M. goes for hemodialysis three days a week at an outpatient clinic in Toronto, taking a small dosage of insulin on dialysis days. He mentioned that before he started dialysis treatment, he had had no appetite for an entire year. After dialysis treatment, he stated that he felt weak and sometimes experienced severe headaches. But his headaches depend on his blood pressure levels. His blood pressure sometimes decreases to 75/40 or 80/40 after hemodialysis, and he often experiences an overall unwell feeling after the treatment.

J.M. stated that his diet is crucial to his health and he follows a strict kidney, healthy heart and diabetic diet. His ability to travel is limited because he is unable to leave the country for any prolonged period, due to his need for hemodialysis treatment. J.M. is on the kidney transplant waiting list. He is hoping that a donor kidney for transplantation will be available for him soon.

Despite his health condition, J.M. said he is blessed. His family plays a big role in his life and they are extremely supportive.

Janice: A New Diagnosis of Hypertension and Kidney Failure

Janice was a 46-year-old African American female who had pursued a career in chiropody. In October 2014, she went to the hospital because she was feeling unwell, had a terrible headache and was urinating frequently. The doctor diagnosed her with high blood pressure and irreversible kidney disease. The doctor also told her that she would need dialysis treatment three days a week. Janice said she had not been aware she even had high blood pressure.

I asked Janice how she was coping, and she said "I am taking it one day at a time." I told her I would be there to provide support and help her cope with her new diagnoses. I also offered to go with her for the initial dialysis consultation visit. I told Janice that she gave me more strength and motivation for writing this book to increase public awareness of hypertension.

I continued to communicate with Janice as I normally would. I left a message for her, and she called back the second week of November 2014. I spent some time with her on the telephone and I asked her how she was feeling. She said she was not doing too badly. I asked her about her follow-up appointment regarding the dialysis. She said the doctor had told her that her kidneys were functioning at only 17 percent, and she would have to reach full kidney failure before she could start dialysis therapy, which could take up to one year.

She said she was still urinating but only small, small amounts each time, and frequently. We chatted about different things. She asked how far along I was with my book and said she was very proud of me. I told her I would call to let her know when I would be visiting, so we could go out before Christmas.

On Monday, November 24, 2014, around 5:25 a.m. my telephone rang. When I answered it, the person on the other end was crying and identified herself as Janice's sister. When I asked what was wrong, she replied, "It is not good. Janice died tragically last night." I was shocked and devastated and could not hold back my tears. She said Janice had had a doctor's appointment the previous week and that her brother had gone with her. At the appointment, Janice was told that she had a heart problem and was given an appointment to see a heart specialist on Tuesday, November 25.

Janice did not get a chance to go to the heart specialist appointment, nor did she get a chance to go for dialysis treatment, because she died Sunday night. A ceremony was held in her memory and a celebration of her life was held in Toronto on November 28 and 29, 2014.

Coping with an illness can be challenging for some people, but coping with multiple chronic diagnoses at the same time can be even more difficult. Therefore, it is important for people, including family members, to recognize individuals who are experiencing difficulty coping with a health condition and provide support to help them cope and manage their illnesses.

Donald's Story

When people are diagnosed with high blood pressure, the experience can be life changing and the impact devastating.

Upon diagnosis, they are usually given the relevant information by their family doctor regarding what their medication will be and the proper dosages. In addition, their doctor will inform them of the changes they have to make with respect to their diet. For example, some foods are good in moderation, some in minimal quantities, and some foods, such as those high in sodium, need to be cut out altogether.

In 2006, I visited my doctor for a physical. He informed me that I was suffering from hypertension. This was nerve-wracking for me. However, my doctor explained the illness to me in great detail. He also said that if I was compliant about my medication and followed a strict and proper diet, which included the relevant food groups that were healthy for my condition, I could live a fairly normal life.

It was June 2006 when I was diagnosed, and my doctor prescribed a blood pressure medication called Diovan. I was required to take one tablet every day, and I followed up with my doctor every three months to make sure my blood pressure was being controlled.

Everything was going well for me for about a year, but in the fall of 2007, during a visit with my doctor, he informed me that my blood pressure was unusually high and that it was in my best interest for him to increase my medication. An additional medication, Adalat, was prescribed for me. So now I was taking one Diovan tablet and one Adalat tablet every day.

I was very disciplined with my medication. After three months, I went to see my doctor again and was elated when he told me that my blood pressure had improved enormously. He said the new medication combination seemed to be working very well.

The information I received from my doctor motivated me so much that I was determined to make sure my blood pressure was kept under control. I took my medication as required, and I was more careful with respect to my diet, reducing my sodium intake dramatically. I also consumed fewer alcohol beverages.

After subsequent visits to my doctor over a period of a year, I realized that the changes I'd made in my lifestyle and my compliance with my blood pressure medications were working very well for me. My doctor was pleased with my progress, and he told me to continue to be vigilant with my health because I was doing so well.

After this, I continued to receive very positive reviews during my doctor visits. My blood pressure remained under control. In September of 2010, during one of my appointments, my doctor told me that he was going to reduce my blood pressure medication to only one prescription. My blood pressure was now well controlled and one tablet daily would be enough for my present condition. Now I only had to take Adalat.

This is a very sobering time in my life, given the positive effects my lifestyle changes are having on my illness. I feel so energized, knowing that I am healthy and am living a normal life. I have been taking only one tablet for my blood pressure for four years now, and my visits to my doctor have been going very well.

I continue to try my best to maintain a healthy diet. I also exercise on a regular basis and remain disciplined with my medication. I am optimistic, knowing that I can live a relatively normal life, even though I have high blood pressure.

10

Hypertension: Prevalence, Consequences and Lifestyle Modification Factors

Hypertension Prevalence in Football Players

The prevalence of hypertension is reported to be high even in athletes. For instance, Karpinos, Roumie, Nian, Diamond and Rothman (2013) stated that a study of professional athletes found National Football League players' prevalence of hypertension was higher when compared to men of the same age in the U.S. population. Karpinos et al. (2013) intended to determine the prevalence of hypertension among collegiate football athletes. They also compared the prevalence of hypertension among this group with nonfootball athletes during their collegiate athletic participation. In addition, the researchers compared the change in college football players' systolic blood pressure to that of nonfootball athletes throughout participants' collegiate career.

Of a total of 636 male participants in the study, 323 were football players and 313 were nonfootball athletes, their sports including football, soccer, baseball, cross-country and basketball. Most activities were offered throughout the year, with the exception of soccer.

In terms of demographic characteristics, football players were likely black, their initial BMI was higher, they had a family history of hypertension and their parental incomes were lower compared to nonfootball athletes.

The study found that the prevalence of hypertension in the initial participation year for football players was 19.2 percent, and it was the same in the final year of their participation. However, compared to nonfootball athletes, football athletes tended to have a higher prevalence of hypertension in the first and final year. For example, it was 19.2 percent for football athletes in the initial year compared to 7.0 percent for nonfootball athletes. In the final year it was

19.2 percent for football athletes compared to 10.2 percent for nonfootball athletes.

The researchers also found that 76 percent of all the athletes in college had either prehypertension or hypertension. Additionally, the prevalence of hypertension was similar in football linemen when compared with those who were not linemen. The results also showed that the prevalence of hypertension was greater in collegiate football athletes compared to the low prevalence of 2.2 percent in male individuals 18 to 24 years old, and 9.1 percent in males 20 to 34 years of age in the U.S. general population.

The findings suggest the necessity for tighter blood pressure screening in communities, not only for football players but for all young men. This is especially so for those with a family history of hypertension and individuals with other risk factors, such as a high BMI. Screening for high blood pressure is especially a priority for African American men. It is estimated that 45 percent of African American people have high blood pressure and 49.9 percent of African American men die from the disease (Bennett, 2013). Similarly, adult African Americans are reported to "have among the highest prevalence of hypertension (44 percent) in the world" (Go et al., 2014, p. 401). Special attention should focus on screening people between 18 and 34 years of age. It is also well known that elevated blood pressure is a risk factor for cardiovascular and kidney morbidity and mortality (Koliaki & Katsilambros, 2013). Therefore, screening people for prehypertension and high blood pressure should be a priority, particularly for African American people. Nevertheless, further research is needed to determine those factors that predispose physically active athletes to prehypertension and hypertension.

Prehypertension and Hypertension: Physical Therapists' Involvement

Physical therapists' early assessment interventions may play a significant role in preventing cardiovascular disease resulting from hypertension. They are able to spot people with prehypertension and hypertension early and refer them for treatment. Arena, Drouin, Thompson, Black and Peterson (2014) determined the prevalence of prehypertension and hypertension blood pressure readings among subjects who were managed by physical therapists in the home care setting. The authors also sought to determine whether there were significant differences in the prevalence of prehypertension and hypertension based on the presence or absence of a known hypertension diagnosis.

The authors reviewed subjects' charts to gather their data on blood pressure readings. It is important to note that only individuals who were managed by physical therapists in the home care setting and had their initial evaluation data entered into electronic health record charts were studied. Chart reviews were performed in three phrases during a six-month accrual period to determine chart eligibility. In phase one review, 763 charts were identified. Of this number, 101 had met the criteria for phase two review. After phase three review, 80 charts had met the study criteria, and these charts were included in the study analyses.

The study subjects consisted of black African Americans, whites, and one American Indian/Alaskan Native subject, as well as participants with unspecified ethnicity. Subjects' mean age was 71, but subjects in their 80s constituted 30 percent of those studied. A larger percentage of study subjects were women (60 percent). White subjects constituted a larger percentage of study subjects (60 percent), versus blacks (21.2 percent) and one American Indian/Alaskan Native subject, with information on ethnicity unavailable for the remaining subjects.

The researchers found prehypertension and hypertension blood pressure readings in 75 percent of studied subjects. For example, prehypertension blood pressure readings were noted in 21 men, an alarming 65.6 percent, whereas 30 women (62.5 percent) had P-HTN blood pressure readings. Women had a higher prevalence of hypertensive blood pressure readings, but their prevalence in the normotensive category was lower.

The study also revealed that 33 subjects (43.1 percent) had known hypertension, while 47 subjects (58.8 percent) had not had a hypertension diagnosis. But the researchers did not find a significant difference in the prevalence of prehypertension and hypertension blood pressure readings that were based on the presence or absence of a known hypertension diagnosis. Of 33 subjects, 31 were known to have hypertension, and they were prescribed medications. The medications were antihypertensive cardiovascular agents.

In terms of ethnic categories, prehypertension was documented in 13 black subjects (76.6 percent), whereas 30 white subjects (57.7 percent) were prehypertensive. It was also shown that six white subjects and one black subject had hypertension readings.

The findings showed that 8.5 percent of subjects who were not diagnosed with hypertension had hypertension blood pressure reading. Arena et al. (2014) concluded that their study is supported by the standards set out for physical therapists, which require them to do cardiovascular screenings when they examine patients. This is to ensure "optimal patient outcomes" (Arena et al., 2014, p. 22).

The findings suggest the need for heightened awareness regarding hypertension prevention at the government level. It is important that policy planners and epidemiologists assess and address community needs to determine contributing factors that put people at risk for diseases such as hypertension. They need to ensure that mandatory policies and guidelines for blood pressure screening are implemented in community settings to inform and increase awareness of the significance and rationale of blood pressure screening. Because this disease is one of the most frequently observed chronic conditions in the primary care setting, and it affects approximately one-third of adult people in the United States (Gallagher, Muntner, Moise, Lin, & Kronish, 2015), education regarding hypertension prevention and control is vital. Hypertension awareness, management and prevention should be promptly addressed to decrease its prevalence and improve people's health. This is important because it is estimated that 25 percent of adults worldwide are affected with hypertension, and the prevalence of the disease is predicted to rise by 60 percent by 2025, when 1.56 billion people will have hypertension (Koliaki & Katsilambros, 2013).

Primary prevention strategies are of uttermost importance to prevent prehypertension in the population and to prevent the onset of cardiovascular illnesses. People with prehypertension are at greater risk of developing hypertension later in their lives (Robbins et al., 2013; Koliaki & Katsilambros, 2013), and are more likely to develop cardiovascular disease than those who are normotensive (Koliaki & Katsilambros, 2013). Koliaki and Katsilambros (2013) also pointed to the high risk factors for cardiovascular and renal illnesses and death related to elevated blood pressure levels. They stated that primary or essential hypertension is the cause of 95 percent of all the cases, and the prevalence is greater in black people of African American descent.

This statistic calls for early and frequent screening for prehypertension and high blood pressure, especially in high risk groups, so people will learn of their diagnoses of prehypertension or hypertension early. As a result, they may change their behavior by implementing meaningful daily lifestyle changes. A change in their lifestyle would likely result in decreasing high blood pressure prevalence in the population and improving blood pressure management. When people take an interest in their health and are motivated to instill positive lifestyle changes, their overall health can improve.

High Blood Pressure in Blacks

Ferdinand and Townsend (2012) state that even though continuing improvements have been made in blood pressure control rates, control is still more likely to be suboptimal in black people than in other racial or ethnic groups. They further reported that this specific group in the United States has an excess of cardiovascular illnesses and death, compared to their white counterparts. Further, Ferdinand and Townsend (2012) report that several factors have been associated with hypertension in the U.S. black population: obesity, especially in women; excess salt intake, coupled with sensitivity to salt; lower intake of dietary potassium; alcohol intake in an excessive amount; and not enough dietary intake of fruits and vegetables.

Target organ damage is also a well-known consequence of hypertension, and since black people tend to develop the disease at an earlier age than white people (Ferdinand & Townsend, 2012), it would be worthwhile to implement early preventive strategies to increase awareness of the effects of hypertension. Primary prevention strategies such as blood pressure screening, decreasing salt intake, increasing fruit and vegetables consumption, decreasing weight, and regular exercise should be stressed to prevent prehypertension and hypertension. The focus of primary prevention measures should target younger black people starting from early teenage years. This population would likely benefit from the interventions because they would be screened for prehypertension and hypertension at an earlier age, and their knowledge would increase if they are given educational material to guide their daily lives and to help them make better lifestyle choices. If this population is properly screened and guided to make healthier choices, prehypertension and hypertension could be detected early and hypertension complications could be decreased. Lives could be saved worldwide.

Additionally, people with known hypertension diagnoses should practice healthy lifestyle behaviors in combination with their prescribed treatment regimen to ensure effective blood pressure control and management. It is also important for educators to be aware and sensitive regarding the material they provide their audience, whether the material is presented in written or oral format. They also need to understand that patients' learning needs and knowledge gaps may vary. It is also important for educators to present the content in a way that is positive, and allow for questions and provide positive feedback. Similarly, educators should understand that individuals are unique in their cultural values and beliefs. As a result, a nonjudgmental teaching approach would probably be more effective, and people may be more attentive and optimistic about learning. People need to know that others care about their health and well-being, and that they are valuable regardless of their health or socioeconomic conditions.

The introduction and implementation of community prevention strategies for blood pressure control in schools, churches, barber shops and community centers in the United States starting at an early stage are mandatory. As such, prehypertension and hypertension could be detected, minimized or prevented. Also, long-term debilitating effects of hypertension consequences, for example, stroke, cardiovascular disease, kidney disease and even death, could be decreased or avoided.

Question: Self-Report Questionnaires for Antihypertensive Medication Adherence

A recent study by Gallagher et al. (2015) examined the properties of the Morisky Medication Adherence Scale (MMAS-8) self-report questionnaire and the Visual Analog Scale (VAS) to identify antihypertensive medication nonadherence in patients whose hypertension was uncontrolled. These methods were compared to electronic measurement, considered the gold standard.

Subjects enrolled in this study were from two hospital–based primary care practices in New York City. These practices were situated in low-income, racially and ethnically diverse neighborhoods. The study consisted of 149 subjects who spoke English or Spanish and had uncontrolled hypertension.

In order to monitor subjects' medication adherence, subjects were given a four-compartment MedSignals pillbox at a routine clinic visit. This pillbox could monitor up to four medications. Every time the lid of the subject's pillbox compartment was opened or closed, the device was able to record that a pill had been taken. Subjects returned the electronic pillbox at the second study visit, and at this time they completed a single MMAS-8 and VAS self-report questionnaire. This questionnaire queried subjects' adherence to all of the antihypertensive medication they took since they last visited the clinic. The MMAS-8 contained six items that assessed the extent of nonadherence and reasons for nonadherence. The score for the questionnaire was measured from zero to eight with eight being the highest adherence. A score less than six was low adherence, less than eight meant medium adherence, and eight showed high adherence.

The VAS has "numbered lines with intervals of 10 percent from 0 to 100 percent for each of the electronically monitored medications" (Gallagher et al., 2015, p. 2). When subjects took each medication, they marked an "X" on the line that corresponded to subjects' estimated adherence while they were being monitored throughout the study. The VAS scores ranged from 0 to 100 percent; a VAS score of 100 percent meant the highest adherence.

It is important to report that subjects' blood pressures were not controlled. At the first clinic visit, the mean systolic blood pressure and diastolic blood pressure were shown to be 159 (19) mm Hg and 85 (12) mm Hg respectively. For most subjects, blood pressures were still not controlled at the second clinic visit, when mean systolic and diastolic readings were reported as 149 (21) mm Hg and 81 (12) mm Hg respectively.

The researchers found that the MMAS-8 and VAS were moderately useful in differentiating between adherent and nonadherent subjects in comparison with the gold standard of electronic measurement. MMAS-8 scores were less than six in 23 subjects, while VAS was less than 80 percent in nine subjects. However, self-report scores that indicated the highest adherence (MMAS-8 = 8) were shown in 43 percent of subjects, whereas VAS scores were 100 percent in 61 percent of subjects.

Gallagher et al. (2015) reported several strengths of their findings. One of the most significant was that the MediSignals pillbox allowed them to measure adherence "to all or most (up to four)" (p. 5) of the subjects' antihypertensive medications instead of monitoring one medication as a surrogate for the total regimen. Another strength was that enrolled subjects were from a diverse limited-income background, as shown by the high proportion of subjects on Medicaid health plans. The authors also believe that their results showed that measuring adherence objectively may be of necessity in guiding clinicians' management of uncontrolled hypertension.

Cardiovascular Disease

Cardiovascular disease due to hypertension is well documented. For instance, Arena et al. (2014) states that "hypertension is a predisposing factor for cardiovascular diseases including congestive heart failure" (p. 18). In black people, high blood pressure is believed to be the main reason and independent risk factor for greater severity of cardiovascular and kidney conditions, as well as stroke and LV hypertrophy, which leads to heart failure and end stage renal disease, resulting in dialysis therapy (Ferdinand & Townsend, 2012).

It is important to recognize and address environmental and individual factors that put people at risk for cardiovascular disease. This is vital because not only does cardiovascular disease impact the individual, but also the strain on the health care system can be enormous. For example, Go et al. (2014), in their report on heart disease and stroke statistics in the United States, reported that "the total number of inpatient cardiovascular operations and procedures increased 28 percent, from 5,939,000 in 2000 to 7,588,000 in 2010" (p. 401). In the United States the combined direct and indirect cost of stroke and cardiovascular disease (CVD) in 2010 was an estimated $315.4 billion. Further, when it comes to diagnostic groups, the researchers also stated that CVD costs more (Go et al., 2014). These statistics suggest a grave need to control the prevalence of CVD in the United States, to help reduce health care costs and improve overall population health.

Robbins et al. (2013) state that it is important to identify early the precursors of chronic disease in people for preconception care and the prevention of adverse consequences of pregnancy. The authors report that identifying CVD risk factors and providing people with information and interventions could improve the health of women of reproductive age, as well as their pregnancy outcomes.

The researchers state that knowledge is partially responsible for reducing chronic disease prevalence and the related CVD risk factors in reproductive-age women with low incomes. Robbins et al. (2013) outline chronic diseases and their precursors as "hypertension, diabetes, and high cholesterol, their precursors (prehypertension, borderline high cholesterol, and prediabetes), and related CVD risk factors such as obesity and smoking" (p. 315).

Robbins et al. (2013) assessed the prevalence of chronic disease, chronic disease precursors and related CVD risk factors among 462 of 859 family planning female patients 18 to 34 years of age who attended a Title X clinic during 2011 and 2012 in eastern North Carolina. Patients were of different races and ethnicities, including 126 white non–Hispanics, 291 black non–Hispanics, 38 Hispanics, and 7 others. The researchers obtained patients' data through self-administered questionnaires that included self-reported current medications patients took for hypertension, diabetes and high cholesterol. Data were also obtained through clinical measurement such as blood pressure readings and BMI. Blood test results, such as cholesterol levels, were also gathered.

The study revealed that of the 462 patients that participated in the study, a vast majority were from minority racial or ethnic groups. For example, black patients represented 63.0 percent of participants and Hispanic, 8.2 percent. It was shown that among these low-income patients, four out of five had one CVD risk factor, and approximately one in three patients had each risk factor, such as prediabetes, prehypertension, smoking and obesity. The prevalence of hypertension was reported to be 11.9 percent, prehypertension 35.1 percent, diabetes 2.6 percent and prediabetes 31.0 percent. The researchers found many patients with newly discovered chronic diseases. For instance, 34 of 54 patients with hypertension, 9 out of 12 patients with diabetes, 138 of 143 patients with prediabetes and 23 patients of 28 with high cholesterol were newly identified.

Of interest, more than a third of the patients were students who were attending either high school or college. Similarly, 97.4 percent of those were either uninsured or publicly insured, and almost all patients reported that the Title X clinic was their only health care source for preventive care.

The findings also show the prevalence of other CVD risk factors in patients. These were obesity, being not physically active or not sufficiently active, and lack of intake of more than five fruits or vegetables daily. It was noted that 70.4 percent of patients were not eating more than five fruit or vegetable servings daily. Also, greater than half of the patients who were considered obese or extremely obese had prehypertension or prediabetes. Prehypertensive patients were less physically active compared to those who were normotensive. Smoking was reported to be high in women who were prediabetic, an alarming 75.2 percent compared to women who were not prediabetic (63.8 percent).

These findings reiterate the grave need to address disparity in U.S. underserved low-income women, especially those of reproductive age, since proper nutrition is vital for women of child-bearing age. Government agencies play a crucial role in addressing the disproportionately low income levels in this group and the decreasing accessibility of health care facilities to optimize health. Interventions and education are meaningful strategies to increase awareness of the importance of adequate nutrition, including the daily recommended intake of fruits and vegetables. Motivating people to adapt meaningful lifestyle changes to improve their behavior and health could be effective if people are given the tools to guide them. Additionally, the government's role is to investigate socioeconomic factors that contribute to unhealthy behavior and poor health outcomes. People have the option to make positive and healthy lifestyle choices to ensure optimal health, but many will require assistance.

Income and education levels are factors that may intervene when people attempt to make decisions and carry out interventions to lead healthier lives. Government agencies can contribute by ensuring that health care needs are addressed, as well as environmental conditions that put people at risk for illnesses and diseases. Policy planners can assist by assessing, planning and implementing accessible community resources for people of low income levels where they can access healthy food at a reasonable cost and alternate health care. Because these factors may improve the health of people and communities, the interventions could be of great benefit in decreasing and preventing illnesses and diseases, possibly reducing health care expenditures.

Proper nutrition is vital not only for women of reproductive age. According to Neville (1987), all people require the same nutrients throughout their lifetime, but the amount varies in a predictive pattern; for instance, "growth, basal metabolic needs, and physical activity are the major factors responsible for changing nutrient needs" (Neville, 1987, p. 1425).

Braunstein, Sherber, Schulman, Ding and Powe (2008) conducted a multicenter cross-sectional study on African Americans and white participants 18 years and older from 13 Maryland outpatient cardiology and general medicine clinic sites between April and October 2002. Patients who had scheduled appointments with a provider at the clinics were eligible for the study. The researchers examined the difference between African American and white participants' perceptions of the risks and benefits of participating in a clinical trial and distrust toward medical researchers, and whether these perceptions influence their willingness to participate in a clinical drug trial. The study utilized a self-administered survey to elicit participants' willingness to participate in a clinical drug trial. Of the eligible participants, 717 took part in the study. Whites constituted 64 percent and African Americans 36 percent of participants.

The results show that 70 percent of participants had responded to the survey. African Americans were likely younger than their white counterparts, lower in the socioeconomic class, and carried a different insurance type than that of white participants. White participants were frequent users of Medicare, while African Americans were underinsured, which was defined as Medicaid or no insurance. In terms of cardiovascular risk profiles, African Americans' hypertension and diabetes mellitus rates were higher, and they smoked more. Whites tended to have a higher rate of coronary artery disease and hypercholesterolemia.

The study also revealed that African Americans' willingness to join a cardiovascular drug prevention trial was less than whites'. This was shown in 41 percent of African American responses. Participants that perceived their personal health would benefit and the quality of their health would be improved if they were willing to participate were more likely to report their willingness. Further, participants who perceived that they would have a greater chance of harm or injury if they joined were less likely to report a positive willingness.

In terms of racial differences regarding the seven components used to gather participants' responses to medical researcher distrust, it was shown that African Americans reported higher levels of distrust compare to whites. It was revealed that for all the domains tested in the index, they proved "African Americans were more likely to express a negative or guarded ("don't know") response than whites" (Braunstein et al., 2008, p. 5). Almost 25 percent of white and African American participants reported that sometimes they were exposed to unnecessary risks by their doctors. Although participants reported they were willing to participate in clinical trials, African Americans still consistently reported greater overall distrust of medical researchers than their white counterparts. Furthermore, more African Americans than white participants believed that their chance would be greater of experiencing harm or injury if they participated in the trial. For example, 45 percent of African Americans and 22 percent of whites perceived a 60 percent higher chance that harm or injury would be experienced from the adverse effects of study-related drugs.

Braunstein et al. (2008) emphasized that attitudes and perceptions are important in African American willingness to join clinical trials, and factors other than socioeconomic may depict the main reasons for racial enrollment disparities. They state that even after adjustments were considered for medical researcher distrust and perceived chance of harm, the issue of race alone did not have a meaningful impact on willingness to participate. The researchers believe that the greater distrust of medical research and researchers that was expressed by African Americans may be due, in part, to the mistrust both of mainstream society and previous examples of medical research conducted on ethnic minorities that were unethical. One example is the United States Public Health Service observational syphilis study, otherwise known as the Tuskegee study.

The findings suggest a grave need to earn the African American people's trust in the medical system, especially when research is involved. But to gain trust will require enormous effort and education. Regardless, clinical research is needed and should be an ongoing process. Results from research studies are important because they will help to guide health care practitioners in their decisions and to determine the specific drug-related treatment that would benefit people of different ethnicities.

Cardiovascular Disease Risk Factors: Differences in Various Ethnicities in Canada

Chiu, Austin, Manuel and Tu (2010) investigated cardiovascular disease risk factors in people of different ethnic backgrounds in Canada. They examined the prevalence of eight cardiovascular risk factors, heart disease and stroke in four different ethnic groups and compared their findings among these groups. The groups consisted of population-based samples of 154,653 white subjects, 3364 South Asian subjects, 3038 Chinese subjects and 2742 black subjects. Subjects lived in Ontario; their ages were 12 years old and older. The researchers used data from five cross-sectional health surveys, which were carried out between 1996 and 2007. It is important to note that the four groups were a representation of the 2001 Ontario census.

The prevalence of major cardiovascular risk factors was highest among blacks; second-highest, whites; third-highest, Chinese; but it was lowest among South Asians. In terms of hypertension prevalence, blacks had the highest, an alarming 19.8 percent. When compared to other groups, the prevalence of hypertension was 17.0 percent for South Asians, 15.1 percent for Chinese, and it was lowest for whites at 13.7 percent. Further, obesity was highest in whites (14.8 percent), second-highest in blacks (14.1 percent), and lowest in Chinese.

It was noted that the Chinese subjects had the lowest cardiovascular risk factors, as well as the lowest prevalence of heart disease and stroke. But this was not so for South Asian subjects. Their prevalence of heart disease and stroke was higher. Heart disease ranged from 3.2 percent in Chinese subjects to 5.2 percent in South Asian subjects.

Not only was the prevalence of hypertension high in blacks and South Asians, but diabetes was also common among these two ethnic groups. In comparison to white subjects, the prevalence of diabetes was two times higher in blacks, and hypertension prevalence was 44 percent higher. In the same fashion, South Asians were more likely to have diabetes compared to their white counterparts.

Physical activity also played a role in cardiovascular risk factors. For instance, it was reported that black women happen to be less physically active, and they were more obese when compared to the overall population. Women of South Asian and Chinese ethnicity were least likely to participate in physical activity on a daily basic relative to the general population.

When risk factors and disease by age and sex were analyzed, the result showed that white men were the group most likely to smoke and to be obese regardless of age. Similarly, white women's smoking prevalence was higher (25.5 percent) in comparison to women in the other groups. For example, only 4.2 percent of Chinese women ages 20 to 44 smoked. Of interest, the prevalence of diabetes was found to be greater in both South Asian men and women who were younger. This difference was also noted in black women more than their white and Chinese counterparts.

Overall, the findings showed that even though black subjects had higher cardiovascular risk factors than the overall population, their prevalence of heart disease was low. A similarity was also observed in Chinese women in term of physical activity. Despite their lower participation in daily physical activity, "people of Chinese origin had significantly lower levels of most cardiovascular risk factors, heart disease and stroke" (Chiu et al., 2010, p. E305).

Chiu et al. (2010) stated that their findings showed differences in cardiovascular risk profiles in the population of all four ethnic groups in Ontario. Based on these differences, it is the authors' belief that there is a need for program development to address cardiovascular risk prevention. They further stated that programs should be specific to the different ethnic groups. They concluded that strategies should focus on cardiovascular risk factors. Also, the developed strategies should address several factors, for example, diabetes and hypertension prevention for those ethnic groups who are high risk, such as blacks and South Asian people.

The findings suggest the need for health education and awareness about heart disease, diabetes and hypertension, especially for black and South Asian people. The development of programs geared toward primary prevention in communities is necessary. Teaching should focus not only on the importance of physical activity, but also healthier lifestyle interventions. Lifestyle choices such as stress reduction, smoking cessation, weight reduction, and healthier food choices would no doubt help to reduce or prevent cardiovascular disease, hypertension, and diabetes in this vulnerable population. People of the aforementioned ethnicities need to be educated based on their susceptive risk factors. Since the prevalence of obesity is believed to be greater in minority women, those with lower levels of education and low incomes (Lefler & Nuss, 2009), the need to address risk factors is crucial. Obesity is "a major modifiable risk factor for coronary artery disease" (p. 349), and obesity also has been directly linked to death (Leflet & Nuss, 2009).

It is important that an assessment of community needs is performed before implementing any type of program. If an assessment is done to determine needs, programs would probably be more successful. Because Ontario represents a diversity of people and different socioeconomic statuses, it is possible that some people may need assistance and guidance to help them make healthier lifestyle choices. There is also a need to educate white men of all ages about the dangers of smoking and its consequences. White women should also be aware of the impact of smoking on their health. Since "cigarette smokers have a two- to fourfold greater risk of developing CHD, twice the risk of having a stroke and ten times the risk of developing peripheral vascular disease" (McCauley, 2006, p. 117). Further, women who smoke cigarettes are believed to have the most prevalent modifiable risk factor for CHD (Lefler & Nuss, 2009). Additionally, women smokers die 14 years sooner when compared to women who do not smoke (McCauley, 2007). Nevertheless, awareness and measures to decrease obesity and smoking among white men and white women in Ontario is warranted if cardiovascular risk factors are to be decreased or prevented. Similarly, heightened awareness is needed in neighboring countries. This is because "women of ethnic minorities are at a disproportionately higher risk for cardiovascular disease than white women in the United States" (Khare et al., 2009, p. 409).

Women and Coronary Artery Disease

Coronary artery disease risk factors are similar to those of coronary heart disease (CHD). For example, Lefler and Nuss (2009) stated that the risk factors for coronary artery disease are greater in African American women compared to Caucasian women. Additionally, their physical inactivity levels, hypertension, diabetes and obesity rates are higher than those of Caucasian women. The authors further stated that women of minority backgrounds have a higher risk of hypertension, but in African American women it is more pronounced. They stated that often these groups are not aware of their higher risk and misunderstood the correlation between hypertension and CHD. Based on this, women need to be educated to broaden their knowledge about CHD and hypertension risk factors to help them lead healthier lives and prevent heart disease.

Arslanian-Engoren (2011) states that in the United States, approximately eight million women have CHD, and the lives lost in women of every demographic and socioeconomic group were greater than 200,000 in the year 2006. The author further reports that this condition is the largest killer of U.S. women. Arslanian-Engoren (2011) points to risk factors for CHD in women such as their age, racial background and socioeconomic status. It is the author's belief that even though all women are at risk for the disease, as they age their likelihood of death from the condition increases. The author reports that for black women the rate for CHD is higher; also they are most likely to die from the condition.

Arslanian-Engoren (2011) stressed the need for screening for CHD risk factors in all women, because the majority of CHD in this group is preventable. The author outlined some of the comorbid risk factors for CHD in women. They are hypertension, diabetes mellitus, hypercholesterolemia, hyperlipidemia and obesity. The other risk factors cited are believed to be modifiable, for example, lifestyle behaviors such as cigarette smoking, not being physically active and the consumption of a high-fat diet. In addition, Arslanian-Engoren reports that decreasing levels of estrogen and progestin have been implied in speeding up the development of CHD in women who are postmenopausal. In the same fashion, irregular menstrual cycles may also increase women's risk of CHD. For example, older women (average age of 50) who have had a history of irregular menstrual cycles have a 28 percent higher risk for developing CHD than women whose menstrual cycle is regular. Pregnant women with a condition of preeclampsia compounded with hypertension and proteinuria at 20 weeks gestation are also at increased risk for developing the disease (Arslanian-Engoren, 2011).

The data indicate that women should exercise caution, especially if they have health conditions and risk factors for CHD, for example, hypertension. This is because the consequences of hypertension are long-term (Fan et al., 2010). Women without risk factors should be proactive and take interest in their health to decrease their chances of developing the condition. It would be of great benefit for all women to implement healthy lifestyle habits. They can do so by eating more fruits and vegetables, decreasing food high in fat and taking part in regular physical activity. Furthermore, the "National Cholesterol Education Program reported that lowering total blood cholesterol level of people with high blood pressure has been shown to reduce their risk for coronary artery disease" (Fan et al., 2010, p. 139). It is also recommended that adult people 20 years old and older check their cholesterol level approximately every five years to decrease their risk for cardiovascular disease (Fan et al., 2010).

Blood Pressure and Cardiovascular Disease

High blood pressure affects cardiovascular outcomes. Cheng et al. (2013) conducted Atherosclerosis Risk in Communities, a community-based study of middle-aged to elderly men and women who were predominantly black and white. Subjects had no cardiovascular disease at study baseline and were followed during a period of 20 years. Study subjects consisted of 13,340 in total; 56 percent were women and 27 percent were black. The researchers compared relative contributions of systolic and diastolic blood pressure, pulse pressure, and mean arterial pressure to subjects' risk for CHD stroke, heart failure and all-cause mortality.

Cheng et al. (2013) documented medical events in all risk categories over the study period. They reported 2095 CHD events, 1669 heart failure events, 771 stroke events, and 3016 deaths during 23 years of the study follow-up. Systolic blood pressure created the greatest risk for CHD in subjects who were nonblack, while in black subjects, mean arterial pressure was the greatest contributor to CHD.

In terms of stroke, elevated systolic blood pressure was reported to be the greatest blood pressure risk contributor to incident stroke in subjects who were black and those who were not black. For all-cause mortality, pulse pressure was the strongest predictor overall. Pulse pressure is the difference between the systolic and diastolic blood pressure readings, and a normal reading is 40. An increased or widened pulse pressure was also reported to be the most significant predictor of incident heart failure. Interestingly, systolic blood pressure and pulse pressure presented risk for heart failure in black subjects, but only pulse pressure was shown to be the strongest risk contributor for heart failure in subjects who were nonblack.

Cheng et al. (2013) concluded that a combination of prior reports as well as their overall findings "suggest that conduit artery stiffening, manifesting as elevated pulse pressure, is likely part of the common pathway leading to the development of heart failure in a majority of individuals at risk" (p. 496).

Burla et al. (2014) recruited African American subjects 35 years and older from the emergency department of Detroit Receiving Hospital. Of the 123 randomized subjects, 88 (45 control group and 43 intervention group) took part in the study treatment protocol. And of the 149 screened subjects, 133 had subclinical hypertensive heart disease. The researchers' purpose was to determine the effects of differing blood pressure goals and increasing therapeutic intensity on perceived health status in this group that showed echocardiographic evidence of subclinical hypertensive heart disease. It is important to note that Burla et al. (2014) utilized a short form survey consisting of 36 questions that elicited subjects' perceptions of their functional health and well-being. Their health status was measured at the initial visit, each quarterly visit, and over one year of follow-up. Subjects' blood pressure was also measured at each quarterly visit, which was every three months.

The researchers found that more intensive antihypertensive therapy was not shown to have a negative impact on subjects' perception of their health status. Blood pressure was steadily decreased over three months at the beginning of the study. The reduction in blood pressure was similar in both intervention and control group, but it barely continued after the first three months. Although the change was not significant in eight of the survey scores over a period of time, there was notable decreased health transition in both groups. This decreased health transition was mostly seen in the early part of the study, but it did not seem to change, even after three months of subject visits and after their medication was intensified over time. Also, no effects could be seen on all parameters for the study group, nor there was any change in blood pressure. However, therapeutic intensity score was found to have an independent association with worsening health transition. Alarmingly, this study also showed "a modest association between rising antihypertensive therapeutic intensity and social functioning" (p. 325).

The researchers report that their findings could help educate people by explaining to them that a need for more medication does not mean they are sicker. They also suggest that their findings could be utilized to encourage intensive blood pressure therapy in those patients on subtherapeutic dosages of high blood pressure medications.

Chronic Kidney Disease (CKD)

Magnetic resonance imaging may play a role in the identification of kidney ischemia, and "inhibitors of the renin-angiotensin system are the cornerstones of the treatment of chronic kidney disease patients" (Siddiqi et al., 2014, p. 214). According to Siddiqi et al. (2014), several experimental studies have revealed that the pathogenesis of chronic kidney disease progression and hypertension is kidney ischemia.

The authors pointed to the challenge of distinguishing the early stage of kidney ischemia (restricted blood supply), but they believe that imaging of the kidney can be carried out with blood oxygenation level dependent (BOLD) magnetic resonance imaging (MRI). The technique will be able to check differences in kidney tissue oxygenation within the segments of the kidneys such as the medulla and cortex.

Siddiqi et al. (2014) conducted a feasibility study on ten male patients with CKD and five healthy volunteers that were considered the control subjects. The selected patients had hypertension and stable CKD, while the healthy subjects were nephrology staff physicians who had volunteered for the study. The purpose of the study was to evaluate BOLD signals before and after patients were treated with 300 mg/day aliskiren for at least six weeks. BOLD MRI scans were done on five patients with CKD. This technique was done one hour before and one hour after their acute treatment with 50 mg of oral captopril medication, while healthy patients were scanned before and one hour after their acute treatment with the same dosage of captopril.

Five patients had an MRI scan done before and after they were put on chronic treatment. The treatment was 300 mg of aliskiren daily for approximately six weeks. All subjects who participated in the study had their blood pressure taken before and after their treatment with the RAS inhibitors and before each BOLD MRI session.

Siddiqi et al. (2014) found that there were changes in BOLD signals in patients with CKD who had received acute and chronic treatment with RAS inhibitors. But this was not so for healthy volunteer subjects; RAS inhibitors showed no effect in BOLD MRI signals in these individuals. The BOLD MRI revealed various hypoxia areas, and these changes were noted in those patients who had renal vascular disease.

The investigators determined that their observations "are compatible with the idea that RAS inhibitors improve kidney oxygenation in patients with CKD, especially of the medulla" (Siddiqi et al., 2014, p. 217). As this study showed increase tissue intensity signal (T2*) in the medulla in CKD patients before and after chronic treatment Captopril, and after their acute treatment with the same medication. But the opposite was noted in the cortex. It was shown that the T2* ratio decreased between the cortex and the medulla in those patients with CKD after both chronic and acute treatment. Note that CKD patients' blood pressure decreased with captopril as well as aliskiren medications, but the effect of captopril was absent in healthy volunteers (controls). It is documented that blockade of the renin-angiotensin-aldosterone system is the present and first treatment therapy for people with chronic renal disease (Kramer, van der Meulen Hamming, van Goor, & Navis, 2007). Siddiqi et al. (2014) concluded that the BOLD MRI technique is a new tool; as a result, it needs to be investigated further.

End-Stage Renal Disease: Psychosocial Impact and Knowledge Needs

End-stage renal disease (ESRD) is a chronic condition (Khalil, Daravad, Gamal, Hamdan-Mansour, & Abed, 2012), and the magnitude of the disease burden will be difficult for some people, thus limiting their ability to cope and effectively manage their condition. Khalil et al. (2012) stated that this disease can have an effect on many aspects of the individual, such as mood, behavior, cognition and their health outcomes. The authors further reported that many factors contribute to adherence of diet and fluid. As a result, they believe that patients receiving hemodialysis for their ESRD are prone to numerous psychosocial disturbances that interfere with patients' adherence. Therefore, it is important that people diagnosed with ESRD be educated about their chronic condition. They need to obtain support to assist them in making decisions about treatment options, dietary needs, overall well-being and kidney transplant requirements. These measures would help people who are suffering from this condition live a more fruitful life while they effectively manage a chronic disease like ESRD.

This is because people with ESRD will require dialysis treatment modalities to sustain their lives (Khalil et al., 2012). Also, newly diagnosed ESRD individuals who are unaware of the appropriate treatment choices and dietary adjustments for their condition may struggle to find information. Limited knowledge will affect patients' ability to make the best treatment decisions. Since dialysis replacement therapy consists of either peritoneal or hemodialysis, it is crucial that people are well informed throughout the stages of their illness. Many people with ESRD might be suitable for transplantation, and "transplantation is the best treatment for end-stage renal failure" (Azancot et al., 2014,

p. 537). This is consistent with Moore et al. (2012), who stated that kidney transplant is the choice of treatment for ESRD. Moreover, kidney transplant is known to increase patients' survival and improve their quality of life, and is preferable compared to conventional dialysis therapies (Moore et al., 2012). Regardless, patients who receive renal transplants need to maintain controlled blood pressure levels. Azancot et al. (2014) report that hypertension is associated "with decreased allograft survival, major adverse cardiac events, and poor patient survival" (p. 537) in patients who received renal transplant. Epidemiologic data suggests that controlled blood pressure improves both graft survival and the survival of patients. The management of medication is also an important factor to consider because patients need to take immune-suppressive medications after renal transplantation for the duration of their graft function, and this could be lifelong (Whittaker, Dunsmore, Murphy, Rolfe, & Trevitt, 2012).

Sinasac (2012) stated that quality of life can be affected by dialysis therapies. Therefore, it is important to recognize individuals that present with decreased coping and institute early interventions to help them cope with the stress and effects of nonfunctional kidneys. This author further reports that many factors contribute to quality of life. Some examples are patients travelling for dialysis treatments, time spent getting dialysis treatments, feelings of not being productive on the days they have dialysis, and various symptoms patients experience prior to dialysis and after therapy (Sinasac, 2012). Khalil et al. (2012) also reports that in terms of psychosocial and cognitive variables, symptoms of depression, individuals' perceptions of the benefits of exercise and barriers, as well as perception of social support all may play a role in the prediction of both dietary and fluid nonadherence.

According to Stewart (2013), "the demands of chronic hemodialysis are considered to be the most stressful of all illnesses and treatment regimens and are suggested to influence individual physical and psychosocial construction of sexuality" (Stewart, 2013, p. 1705). The author listed sexual changes that are physically related and psychosocial changes that are believed to be associated with hemodialysis. According to Stewart (2013), physical sexuality changes are erectile dysfunction, which is notable in men, and decreased sexual satisfaction. Psychosocial changes are loss of time and lifestyle changes. In addition, other physical and psychosocial changes are "frequent arterial and venous punctures, pigmentation of the skin and appearance changes, food and fluid restrictions," limitations in physical mobility, altered family role, and "feeling of inadequacy" (Stewart, 2013, p. 1705).

In terms of lifestyle changes and the loss of time, Stewart (2013) stated that an example of a detrimental effect is the amount of time patients on hemodialysis spend in a dialysis environment. This is 3 to 5 hours, three days or more in one week alone.

Nunes et al. (2011) stated that whenever ESRD patients obtain more knowledge about their disease, the knowledge has been linked to increased use of patient-preferred access types for hemodialysis therapy, as well as more participation in self-management behaviors. People with CKD also need education about the disease and its processes. Nunes et al. (2011) reported that patients need education about CKD, education is key part of comprehensive predialysis care, and it has been associated with improved clinical outcomes. Sinasac (2012) states that if improvement is made in managing diabetes mellitus and hypertension, the improvement measures "can significantly prevent the development of CKD" (p. 25), because these conditions are the leading causes of CKD (Sinasac, 2012).

Nunes et al. (2011) examined whether there were associations between objective knowledge and perceived knowledge in CKD. The researchers utilized a kidney disease knowledge survey and a perceived kidney disease knowledge survey in 399 patients at all stages of CKD who were not dialysis dependent. Patients were from various nephrology clinics. Study patients were nonwhite and white and their mean age was 58 years. Forty-seven percent were women, and 77 percent of patients had stages 3 to 5 CKD. A greater percentage of participants were Caucasians (83 percent). The authors further examined their knowledge of patient-perceived knowledge to determine whether there were associations with objective kidney knowledge and patient satisfaction with their provider's interpersonal communication skills.

Regarding objective perceived knowledge of kidney function, the authors concluded that this was limited in patients. For example, greater than 50 percent had reported little or no knowledge about medications that helped the kidney. This was shown in 72 percent of patients. Sixty-three percent reported little or no knowledge about medications that hurt the kidneys. Regarding diet, 63 percent of patients had little or no knowledge about foods they should stay away from if they have low kidney function. Additionally, 51 percent had little or no knowledge regarding the functions of the kidney, and 61 percent reported little or no knowledge of the symptoms of CKD.

Most alarming, 25 percent of patients had reported "that they knew little or nothing about why they were sent to a kidney doctor" (p. 1347), despite the fact that 58 percent of patients had visited a kidney doctor (renal specialist) on at least three occasions in the past year. While 64 percent felt they knew how kidney function was checked by a doctor, 77 percent of patients had a good amount or a lot of knowledge of what their goal blood pressure should be.

When the associations with perceived kidney knowledge were analyzed, the results showed that perceived knowledge was associated with objective knowledge. Also, increasing age was found to be a significant association with decreasing perceived knowledge. Interestingly, variables that showed an independent association with overall perceived kidney knowledge were older age, male gender, higher average glomerular filtration rate (eGFR), nonattendance at CKD class, and health literacy, which was less than ninth grade. Yearly income was also associated with perceived knowledge. For instance, those with income of more than $55,000 a year had a higher perceived knowledge when compared to those with less than $25,000 a year. However, patients' years of education or the amount of visits made to the doctor were not associated with overall perceived knowledge. It was also determined that patients often knew someone else with kidney disease.

A positive relationship was shown between perceived knowledge and satisfaction with provider communication. However, a negative relationship was shown between satisfaction and objective knowledge. For instance, patients who were older, had higher eGFR, and higher perceived knowledge had higher odds of satisfaction regarding communication with their provider. But patient satisfaction with provider communication showed no association with race, health literacy, income, or number of visits to providers. Furthermore, "higher objective knowledge scores were associated with lower odds of satisfaction with provider communication" (Nunes et al., 2011, p. 1347).

The authors emphasized the importance for accurate measurement and clear definition of all types of knowledge in terms of perceived and objective disease knowledge in research studies such as their own study.

In a national population study, Yan et al. (2014) examined all-cause hospitalizations among patients who were receiving long-term hemodialysis, including their hospital days, admission rates, and whether race/ethnicity or age had modified the rates. The authors also examined those rates for three common cause-specific hospitalizations, such as cardiovascular diseases, all-cause infections and dialysis-related infection. The authors utilized the U.S. Renal Data System to identify patients who were over 18 years of age and who were beginning maintenance dialysis for the first time in the United States between April 1, 1995, and June 30, 2009. The study consisted of 563,281 patients of three different racial/ethnic groups. Of these, whites constituted 55.4 percent, blacks 32.7 percent and Hispanics 11.9 percent. Patients were grouped in three age groups at ESRD onset: 18 to 40, 41 to 70 and over 70 years old.

Yan et al. (2014) reported the primary outcomes for patients' total hospital days and admissions per year for all-cause and cause-specific hospitalization, which included cardiovascular diseases, all-cause infection, and dialysis-related infection.

The researchers found that 912,723 hospital admissions occurred, for a total of 7,026,229 hospital days over a median of one year of follow-up. The average rates were 14.95 hospital days and 2.03 admissions per patient annually.

Regarding all-cause hospitalization, it was shown that black and Hispanic rates were lower than white patients. This was evident only in the 51 to 60 and 61 to 70 years age groups. Additionally, all-cause hospitalization was the lowest in Hispanics, intermediate in blacks, and the highest in whites. The authors pointed to the adjusted black-white ratio for hospital days, which demonstrated a U-shaped pattern with age. The highest rate was seen in blacks who were younger than 40 years and those in the older age groups.

In relation to cause-specific hospitalizations, a combination of cardiovascular diseases and all-cause infections were the cause of most hospitalized days and hospital admissions. Also, approximately one-third of all-cause infectious hospitalizations were related to dialysis infections.

There were differences across age groups in all-cause infectious hospitalizations. For instance, younger black patients less than 40 years of age had a greater percentage of all-cause infection compared to whites. Hispanic and black rates of hospitalization were higher than white patients, and these high rates were because of dialysis-related infections. This was consistently noted in all age groups for blacks. The authors reported that although the rates of hospitalization related to cardiovascular diseases increased in patients of older age, hospital rates due to dialysis-related infection moderately decreased with age.

In summary, the study findings revealed that Hispanic patients' all-cause hospital days and hospital admissions rates were lower. In contrast, black patients' all-cause admissions were higher. Age seemed to play a role. For instance, the fewest hospital days as well as admissions were of Hispanic patients in all the age groups younger than 70 years; meanwhile, the highest rates were observed in Hispanic patients over 80 years.

The authors concluded that black and Hispanic people are at greater risk of hospitalization than white people. This may due, in part, to the hospital rates for Hispanics from dialysis-related infection, because after age 80 their rates were higher than whites. Yan et al. (2014) believed that these rates are probably related to lower rates of arteriovenous (AV) fistula placement. The study showed that both black and Hispanic patients were less likely to receive erythropoietin stimulation agents, pre–ESRD nephrologist care, and the use of AV fistula. They also pointed to the need for further studies to comprehensively examine health beliefs and behavior factors, among other variables. They believed the interventions may help to decrease hospital admissions and provide cost-effective measures in people receiving dialysis treatment.

Overview of Vitamin D, Hypertension and Cardiovascular Disease

Vitamin D and Hypertension

Studies have often found that low vitamin D levels have been linked to hypertension (Tamez, Kalim, & Thadhani, 2013), and according to Lavie, DiNicolantonio, Milani, & O'Keefe (2013), "vitamin D plays a substantial role in determining the risk of various metabolic conditions and, particularly metabolic syndrome/type 2 diabetes mellitus and systemic hypertension" (p. 2404). Systemic hypertension refers to hypertension in the systemic arteries and is usually caused by constriction of small arteries (arterioles). Lavie et al. (2013) further state that this vitamin also plays a role in how the renin-angiotensin-aldosterone system (RAAS) is regulated. When there is a deficiency in this vitamin, the RAAS upregulates, predisposing the body to hypertension, including hypertrophy of the smooth muscle cells found in the vascular tree and the left ventricle (Lavie et al., 2013).

One of the mechanism in which vitamin D may have an influence on blood pressure is its power to negatively regulate the RAAS (Motiwala & Wang, 2011). For example, Motiwala and Wang (2011) state that when vitamin D receptors were inactivated in mice, they had increased plasma renin activity and elevated blood pressure; these conditions were reversed with angiotensin-converting enzyme (ACE) inhibitors. The authors believe that the effects of vitamin D on the suppression of renin may be due to direct effects on gene expression. Further, "renin, angiotensin (I and II) and aldosterone play an important role in hypertension and are current targets of medical therapy" (Tamez et al., 2013, p. 497).

Motiwala and Wang (2011) also point to observational studies that revealed an inverse correlation between vitamin D levels and plasma renin activity, as well as many cross-sectional studies that showed "that lower vitamin D levels are associated with higher blood pressure or higher prevalence of hypertension" (Motiwala & Wang, 2011, p. 347). The U.S. National Health and Nutrition Examination Survey (NHANES III) study showed an inverse relationship between mean blood pressure and serum 25 OH Vitamin D levels. The association was significant even after they had adjusted for age, sex, race/ethnicity and physical activity. Tamez et al. (2013) stated that several large cross-sectional studies have shown a strong relationship between a deficiency in vitamin D and an increase in blood pressure, as well as an increased risk of hypertension.

Similarly, Judd, Raiser, Kumari and Tangpricha (2010) conducted a pilot feasibility study examining whether vitamin D lowers blood pressure and plasma renin activity in humans. This study screened a total of 33 participants; nine were enrolled but only seven participated over the three-week study period. Participants were over 30 years of age, African American, and were recruited from the Atlanta Veterans Affairs Medical Center in Decatur, Georgia. Participants' 25 OH Vitamin D levels were between 25 and 75 nmol/L and their systolic blood pressures were between 130 mm Hg and 150 mm Hg. An evaluation of the inactive form of vitamin D, known as cholecalciferol or vitamin D_3, and the active form of vitamin D, called calcitriol, was carried out for the study.

Participants were randomized to receive cholecalciferol, calcitriol or placebo in three groups. They received calcitriol, cholecalciferol, or placebo by mouth. For this study, participants received 200,000 IU of cholecalciferol or matching placebo on a weekly basis for 3 weeks, or 0.5 mg calcitriol twice a day for only one week. Calcitriol was given more frequently because of it short half-life, which is eight hours. Participants continued to take their prescribed blood pressure medication during the study.

The findings show that participants' systolic blood pressure was decreased with calcitriol, the active form of vitamin D, when compared to the placebo. However, there was no notable significant change in participants' systolic pressure with the inactive form of vitamin D, cholecalciferol, when compared to placebo. Participants in the calcitriol group had a 9 percent decrease in systolic blood pressure, but did not experience a significant decrease in their diastolic blood pressure. There was a decrease in their heart rate, and the reduction was found to be significant in comparison to those in the placebo group.

Notably, a significant reduction in blood pressure was seen in one participant with high plasma renin activity who was treated with cholecalciferol. Based on this, the researchers believe that for future studies, cholecalciferol therapy should target people with high plasma renin activity.

The authors also evaluated whether participants' reduction in systolic pressure was sustained at the calcitriol follow-up. This was a week after participants had had calcitriol treatment and had worn ambulatory blood pressure monitors for a week. Judd et al. (2010) found that participants' systolic blood pressure had returned to levels recorded prior to their treatment.

Despite their valuable results, the authors emphasized that data should be interpreted with caution "as calcitriol is a risky antihypertensive therapy" (Judd et al., 2010, p. 447). Also, a larger sample size would be required for future studies to explore its safety and efficacy.

The Adventist Health Study, a cross-sectional study by Sakamoto et al. (2013), was conducted on a random selection of 568 participants, both men and women, age 30 to 95 years. Of this number, 284 were whites and 284 were blacks. The researchers examined whether vitamin D levels of participants with a broad range of dietary patterns were associated with blood pressure in non-Hispanic whites and blacks who generally have healthy lifestyle habits. It is important to note that Seventh–Day Adventists eat a variety of diets, including vegetarian, and the majority of participants did not drink alcohol or smoke.

Sakamoto et al. (2013) found that there was an inverse relationship between serum vitamin D levels and systolic blood pressure in nondiabetic white participants, but the relationship was not shown in black participants. The results were similar in blacks even after age, gender, the use of blood pressure medications, waist circumference, and participants' body fat percentage instead of their BMI levels were all taken into consideration by the researchers. The results showed no relationship between serum 25 OHVitamin D levels and diastolic blood pressure in black participants. The same inverse relationship between 25 OH Vitamin D and systolic blood pressure was observed in whites who were not being treated for hypertension, but there was no significant association among white participants receiving hypertension treatment. However, the relationship was not seen in blacks who were treated for hypertension and those who were not treated for hypertension. Nevertheless, serum 25 OH Vitamin D levels were found to be higher in white participants compared to blacks, and the vitamin D deficiency percentage was higher for blacks (55 percent in blacks versus only 15 percent in whites). In regard to dietary patterns, there was a huge difference between the participants. For instance, blacks had consumed more meat products, whereas whites had consumed more dairy products.

The authors elaborated on the strength of their study, which showed that participants were predominantly nonsmokers, were not alcohol drinkers, and they mainly performed regular physical activity. One benefit of this sample population is that participants reported a broad range of dietary patterns, ranging from pure vegan to omnivore.

Rostand (2010) examined the role vitamin D deficiency may play in the pathogenesis and maintenance of hypertension in African diaspora people. According to Rostand (2010), native Africans and other people of color who live near the equator tend to have a lower prevalence of hypertension in comparison to those people who live at more northern or southern latitudes. They stated that for each ten degrees north or south of the equator, blood pressure increases by 2.5 mm Hg and the prevalence of hypertension increases by 2.5 percent. It is Rostand's belief that "because blood pressure has been shown to vary inversely with UVB light availability and because people of color have a high prevalence of low circulating levels of 25-hydroxyvitamin D_3 [25(OH)D_3], it has seemed reasonable to speculate that vitamin D deficiency may contribute to their increased prevalence of hypertension" (p. 509).

Rein-Angiotensin System and Its Role in Vitamin D

Furthermore, Rostand (2010) believed that hypertension and the upregulation of the RAAS observed in mice with inactive vitamin D receptors may be related to the vascular changes that are noted in African Americans. This is due to the stimulatory effects of vitamin D deficiency and its impact on RAAS. Angiotensin II is believed to upregulate extracellular matrix proteins, including promoting fibrosis of vascular smooth muscle cells, resulting in vascular stiffness. These effects are suppressed by 1, 25 OH Vitamin D_3 by downregulating renin production. The results have allowed the authors to speculate that the vascular changes shown in African Americans may be related to the aforementioned effects.

Rostand (2010) also stated that varying differences exist in African American people and Caucasian people in terms of their microvascular structure and function, such as increased systemic and renal vascular resistance and decreased renal blood flow, which may cause the RAAS to activate. Whenever there is an activation of the RAAS and pro-inflammatory cytokines (immune system chemicals that promote inflammation), the result is vascular endothelial dysfunction and microvasculature structural changes that progress to vascular stiffness and increased resistance. These structural changes have been demonstrated to precede the beginning of hypertension and may happen very early in an individual's life.

These observations of immune system activation support current theories regarding an autoimmune hypertensive syndrome. In the condition of autoimmune hypertension, patients are known to secrete excess catecholamines (epinephrine, norephinephrine), which activate the alpha-adrenergic transduction system. These patients have been found to have autoantibodies to the beta adrenergic receptor. These autoantibodies have previously been found in patients with idiopathic dilated cardiomyopathy, Chagas' disease, and other forms of cardiomyopathy (Kem, et al., 2007; Kalache, 2015).

Vitamin D and Heart Disease

It has been estimated that nearly a billion people worldwide have a deficiency in vitamin D (Tamez et al., 2013). Similarly, Lavie et al. (2013) reported that a deficiency of this vitamin is prevalent in the United States and around the world.

It is reported by Robinson-Cohen et al. (2013) that a low circulation of serum vitamin D has been found to constantly link with an increased risk of clinical and subclinical coronary heart disease (CHD). Robinson-Cohen et al. (2013) conducted the Multi-Ethnic Study of Atherosclerosis on 6436 adult subjects without clinical cardiovascular disease. The purpose of the study was to examine the association of serum 25 OH Vitamin D with risk of CHD to determine if risk differed among white, black, Chinese, and Hispanic subjects. The subjects were 38 percent white, 28 percent black, 22 percent Hispanic, and 12 percent Chinese. Their ages were 45 to 84 years; they were recruited from six field centers in the United States from 2000 to 2002.

The researchers found that mean serum 25 OH Vitamin D concentration was 25.5 (10.6) ng/mL, and the concentration varied by ethnicity. For instance, in white subjects the level was 30.1 (10.6) ng/mL, followed by 26.7 (8.3) ng/mL among Chinese, 19.2 (9.0) ng/mL for blacks and 24.6 (9.4) ng/mL in Hispanics.

In terms of CHD events, there were 361 occurrences by the clinical endpoint. The incidence rate was 7.38 events per 1000 person-years. This was observed during median follow-up of 8.5 years. Lower serum 25 OH Vitamin D concentrations were found to be associated with higher risks of CHD. This was observed in white and Chinese subjects, but no similar association was shown in black and Hispanic subjects. The association differences were consistent across the ethnic groups for a broad and restricted definition of CHD utilized for the study, and remained after adjustments were made for the known risk factors for CHD.

The authors pointed out that further analyses regarding racial differences and the associations of 25 OH Vitamin D with CHD are required to confirm their study findings. Until the study is completed, they emphasized that "results of studies testing associations of circulating 25 OH Vitamin D concentrations with CHD or related outcomes in predominantly white populations should not be extrapolated to multiracial populations" (Robinson-Cohen et al., 2013, p. 283).

Summary

The chapters in this book present a broad view of hypertension, based on an extensive medical literature review. In the earlier chapters, hypertension, its risk factors prevalence, and causes are described in detail. Nonpharmacological management, such as lifestyle changes, and pharmacological management for hypertension control and management are extensively summarized. I have reported research findings that emphasized the grave need to effectively control and manage hypertension in the population to decrease hypertension prevalence, decrease and prevent its potential complications, and decrease death rates worldwide. Greater emphasis is given to black people due to their higher prevalence of the disease and adverse effects of hypertension at an early stage.

The text also stresses the significance of screening for high blood pressure, primary preventive measures and education. The involvement of policy planners in implementing strategies to increase awareness of prehypertension and hypertension is needed. Addressing socioeconomic factors related to the existing disparities, especially in the African American community, is a priority.

Although some people with hypertension may face obstacles in modifying their diet and lifestyle, they should make an effort to change their behavior to lead a healthier life and decrease their risk of developing complications due from hypertension. People with a chronic disease like hypertension may find it difficult to cope; as a result, they can seek support from family, friends or their health care providers. This is because chronic disease can be a challenge to live with daily, and some people may require support to effectively cope with a long-term illness such as hypertension. Further, people with hypertension need to adopt dietary changes that require commitment and discipline. How people react to life and environmental changes will definitely play a significant role in their ability to cope, control and manage their health condition.

My hope is that readers will find the information in these chapters useful, guiding them and helping them prevent, control, and manage hypertension. Nevertheless, further research is necessary worldwide. In the United States, more research is needed on African American people regarding hypertension control and their views about hypertension control and management. Research should also focus on younger African American men. The whys behind the documented high prevalence and uncontrolled hypertension, especially in African American people, have yet to be determined. Thus, only ongoing research will solve this puzzle and possibly eradicate hypertension in this vulnerable population.

Appendix 1. Sample Five-Day Meal Plan

This menu provides a basic plan with foods from all food groups, such as protein, grains, fruits, vegetables, milk and cheese products. It is specifically designed for people with high blood pressure. Omitting or decreasing salt in your diet is imperative for blood pressure control and management.

It is important to note that your daily intake will be based on your caloric needs and whether weight reduction is your goal. It is recommended that individuals consult their doctors before starting any new diet, especially if they are allergic to certain foods.

Try to eat at the same time every day, if possible.

Invest in measuring utensils and keep them within reach for cooking. They will help you accurately measure food items until you feel comfortable preparing meals without using them. Measuring utensils can be purchased for a low cost at discount or dollar stores.

BASIC METRIC MEASUREMENT CONVERSIONS

1 teaspoon = 5 mL; 1 tablespoon = 15 mL; ¼ cup = 60 mL; ½ cup = 120 mL; 3/4 cup = 180 mL; 1cup = 240 mL

Day One

***Breakfast:** 7 a.m.*

1 cup rolled oats

¼ teaspoon cinnamon

½ teaspoon grated nutmeg

½–1 cup 1 percent milk (If lactose intolerant, try lactose-free milk.)

Optional: 1 tablespoon of sugar can be added for additional flavor, if you're nondiabetic.

In medium pot, bring 2 cups of water to a boil. Add oats and stir until smooth.

Add cinnamon, nutmeg, milk, and stir. Boil over medium heat for 5 minutes. Remove from heat and allow to cool for 2 to 3 minutes, then enjoy.

Snack: 10 a.m.

½ cup fruit or ½ cup plain yogurt

Lunch: 12:30 to 1 p.m.

2½ ounces skinless chicken breast

1 cup steamed mixed vegetables

½–1 cup parboiled rice

Season chicken breast with ½ cup chopped onion, 3 cloves finely chopped garlic, 1 small diced tomato, 1 teaspoon black pepper, and 1 teaspoon paprika. Mix together ¼ cup water with 2 tablespoons olive oil and add to a pan, along with the chicken and seasonings. Cover and oven boil at 300°F for 45 to 50 minutes or until cooked through but tender.

Snack: 3:30 to 4 p.m.

⅓ cup unsalted almonds

Dinner: 6:30–7:30 p.m.

2½ ounces lean meat

1 medium-sized baked sweet potato

1 cup salad

Season meat with ½ cup chopped onion, 3 cloves finely chopped garlic, 1 small diced tomato, 1 teaspoon black pepper, and 1 teaspoon paprika. Mix together ¼ cup water with 2 tablespoons olive oil and add to a pan, along with the meat and seasonings. Cover and oven boil at 300°F for 45 to 50 minutes or until cooked through but tender.

Snack: 8 p.m.

1 triangle Laughing Cow cheese

Try this: Place 3 to 4 slices of cucumber in 1 cup water for flavor. You can drink this instead of sodas.

Day Two

Breakfast: 7 a.m.

2 slices multigrain bread, toasted

1 boiled egg

1 cup green tea

Optional: Add 1 teaspoon sugar and 1 tablespoon 1 percent milk, if desired, to tea. Diabetics may refrain from adding sugar.

Snack: 10 a.m.

½ cup blueberries

Lunch:* 12:30–1 *p.m.
1 small can low-salt salmon
lemon juice, to taste
black pepper, to taste
½ cup bulgur
1 cup steamed spinach
To a small saucepan, add ¼ cup water, spinach, 1 teaspoon olive oil, ½ cup chopped onions, 1 small diced tomato, 1 teaspoon black pepper, 1 teaspoon paprika. Steam on stove over low heat for 10 to 15 minutes. Season with lemon juice and additional black pepper, if desired.

Snack:* 3:30–4 *p.m.
1 medium-sized banana

***Dinner:* 6:30–7:30**
½–¾ cup dried lentils
1 medium-sized baked Yukon potato
½–1 cup mixed steamed vegetables
Soak lentils overnight in a bowl of water. When ready to cook, drain lentils, then place them in a pot with enough water to cover. Bring to a boil, and simmer until tender.

Snack:* 8 *p.m.
1 medium-sized nectarine or apple

Day Three

Breakfast:* 7 *a.m.
1 cup Red River cereal
½–1 cup 1% milk
¼–½ teaspoon grated nutmeg
¼ teaspoon cinnamon
½ cup frozen berries, thawed
Optional: Nondiabetics can add 1 to 2 teaspoons sugar, if desired, keeping in mind that the berries provide natural sweetness.
To a pot, add the cereal, nutmeg, cinnamon, and 2 cups of water. Stir until smooth. Bring to a boil. Decrease heat to medium. Add milk and cook mixture for 15 to 20 minutes, or until grains are tender. Mix in berries. Let cool for 3 to 5 minutes, then savor.

Snack:* 10 *a.m.
½ cup blueberries or strawberries

Lunch: 12:30–1 p.m.
1 or 2 slices multigrain bread
2 tablespoons peanut butter
1 cup salad, which can include a mixture of leafy green romaine lettuce, deep orange, red and yellow peppers, cucumber, and tomatoes.

Snack: 3:30–4 p.m.
⅓ cup nuts, unsalted. (Try lower-fat nuts whenever possible.)

Dinner: 6:30–7:30 p.m.
2½ ounces snapper (fish)
½–1 cup parboiled rice
1 cup steamed or boiled okra (8 pieces), or mixed vegetables
Season snapper with ½ cup chopped onion, 3 cloves finely chopped garlic, 1 small diced tomato, 1 teaspoon black pepper, and 1 teaspoon paprika. Mix together ¼ cup water with 2 tablespoons olive oil and add to a pan, along with the snapper and seasonings.
Cover and steam on stove over low to medium heat for approximately 45 minutes. Serve snapper over rice, alongside okra.

Snack: 8 p.m.
½ cup plain yogurt

Day Four

Breakfast: 7 a.m.
1 to 2 slices multigrain bread, toasted
1 slice low-salt Swiss cheese
2 slices tomato, 3 slices cucumber, lettuce
1 cup tea, plain or with 2 teaspoons of 1% milk

Snack: 10 a.m.
⅓ cup nuts, unsalted

Lunch: 12:30–1 p.m.
½–1 cup quinoa, cooked according to package directions
3 ounces halibut or sole
½ cup steamed vegetables
Season halibut or sole with 1 tablespoon olive oil, ¼ cup chopped onions, 1 small diced tomato, and 3 cloves finely chopped garlic. To a saucepan, add ¼ cup water and the seasonings. Add fish. Cover and steam on stove for 25 to 30 minutes, or to your liking. Serve fish over quinoa, alongside vegetables.

Snack: 3:30–4 p.m.
½ cup grapes

Dinner: 6:30–7 p.m.
3 ounces turkey breast
1 cup salad
½–1 cup cooked whole wheat pasta
In a baking tray, season turkey with 2 tablespoons olive oil, ¼ cup chopped onions, 1 small diced tomato, 3 cloves finely chopped garlic, 1 teaspoon paprika, ½ teaspoon black pepper, and a squeeze of lemon juice. Cover turkey and bake at 300°F for 40 to 45 minutes.

Snack: 8 p.m.
1 small glass orange juice

Day Five

Breakfast: 7 a.m.
1 or 2 eggs, fried
2 slices multigrain bread, toasted
2 slices tomato, 3 slices cucumber, lettuce
Combine the ingredients to make a delicious sandwich.

Snack: 10 a.m.
1 triangle Laughing Cow cheese

Lunch: 12:30–1 p.m.
2 slices whole wheat bread
4 ounces low-salt canned tuna
½–1 cup cut-up, raw vegetables
¼ cup finely chopped onions
½ small diced tomato
¼ teaspoon mayonnaise (if desired)
¼ teaspoon black pepper
Add lemon juice to taste
Mix tuna and other ingredients together. Combine with bread and vegetables to make a delicious sandwich.

Snack: 3:30–4 p.m.
½ cup fruit

Dinner: 6:30–7:30 p.m.
1 medium-sized sweet potato, baked
1 cup salad

½–1 cup dried beans and/or lentils

Soak lentils overnight in a bowl of water. When ready to cook, drain lentils, and then place them in a pot with enough water to cover. Bring to a boil, and simmer until tender. Add 1 tablespoon unsalted butter for extra flavor.

Snack: 8 p.m.

Small-sized pear or banana

Appendix 2. Test Your Knowledge of Hypertension

These questions were developed to test your awareness of hypertension. The answers follow. Choose either T (true) or F (false). Let's get started!

QUESTIONS

1. If I feel sick, I should not take my blood pressure pills. T or F?
2. I don't have any blood pressure medication to take today, but it's okay to refill it in two days. T or F?
3. My blood pressure pills give me a headache, so to stop taking them is the better choice for me. T or F?
4. Eating a high-fiber diet, one that includes fruits and vegetables and foods low in fat, is good for people with high blood pressure. T or F?
5. Foods high in salt are dangerous for people with high blood pressure. T or F?
6. Walking three times a week, for 30 minutes each time, is good for blood pressure control. T or F?
7. Excess body weight contributes to uncontrolled blood pressure in some people. T or F?
8. Heart disease, kidney disease, and stroke are three major health conditions due, in part, to hypertension. T or F?
9. Hypertension is an acute disease. T or F?
10. People with hypertension usually show symptoms. T or F?
11. Hypertension affects people of all cultural backgrounds. T or F?
12. People should be screened for high blood pressure. T or F?
13. Only older people get high blood pressure. T or F?

14. The prevalence of hypertension is higher in white people than in African American people. T or F?

15. Your doctor is the only person responsible for keeping your blood pressure under control. T or F?

ANSWERS

1. False—Your doctor prescribed your blood pressure medication to control your blood pressure, so you should not skip it. If your medication is making you feel sick, discuss this with your doctor right away.

2. False—If your doctor told you to take your blood pressure medication every day, you should take it every day. Try to refill your prescriptions right away so that you're not caught without your daily medicine.

3. False—Never stop taking your blood pressure medication before first consulting with your doctor.

4. True—Studies show that high-fiber foods, like fruits and vegetables, in combination with blood pressure medication can help control high blood pressure.

5. True—People with high blood pressure should try to avoid high-salt foods.

6. True—Studies show that any form of exercise is good for people with hypertension. Walking is a form of exercise that will help to control blood pressure.

7. True—Studies show that increased body mass index (BMI) has been linked to hypertension and uncontrolled hypertension in some individuals. The maintenance of a BMI of 20 to 25 is recommended (Bunker, 2014).

8. True—Studies continually find that people who suffer from hypertension are at risk for developing these conditions.

9. False—Hypertension is a chronic disease.

10. False—People with hypertension do not show any symptoms.

11. True—People from all cultural backgrounds can develop hypertension.

12. True—It is very important that individuals be screened for high blood pressure.

13. False—While high blood pressure most commonly develops in middle and old age, a study done in 1999 to 2000 found that in people "8 to 17 years old, systolic blood pressure levels were 2.9 and 1.6 mm Hg higher in non–Hispanic black boys and girls, respectively, than in age-matched non–Hispanic whites" (Flack et al., 2010, p. 781). This study shows that younger people can exhibit characteristics of hypertension. Another study found that "one in five

Thai people aged at least 15 years has high blood pressure" (Aekplakorn et al., 2012, p. 1734).

14. False—Several studies have documented that hypertension is more prevalent in African Americans than in whites.

15. False—Hypertensive individuals, in cooperation with their doctors, need to take responsibility and measures to keep their blood pressure under control.

Bibliography

Abeyta, I.M., Tuitt, N.R., Byers, T.E., & Sauaia, A. (2012). Effect of community affluence on the association between individual socioeconomic status and cardiovascular disease risk factors, Colorado, 2007–2008. *Prev Chronic Dis, 9,* 110305. DOI: http://dx.doi.org/10.5888/pcd9.110305.

Aekplakorn, W., Sangthong, R., Kessomboon, P., Putwatana, P., Inthawong, R., Taneepanichskul, S., ... Sritara, P. (2012). Changes in prevalence, awareness, treatment and control of hypertension in Thai population, 2004–2009: Thai National Health Examination Survey III-IV. *J Hypertension, 30*(9), 1734–1742.

Alkadry, M.A., Bhandari, R., Wilson, C.S., & Blessett, B. (2011). Racial disparities in stroke awareness: African Americans and Caucasians. *J Health and Human Services Admin, 33*(4), 462–490.

Allicock, M., Johnson, L., Leone, L., Carr, C., Walsh, J., Ni, A., ... Campbell, M. (2013). Promoting fruit and vegetable consumption among members of black churches, Michigan and North Carolina, 2008–2010. *Prev Chronic Dis, 10,* 120161. DOI: http://dx.doi.org/10.5888/pcd10.120161.

Al-Zahrani, M.S. (2011). Prehypertension and undiagnosed hypertension in a sample of dental school female patients. *International J Dental Hygiene, 9*(1), 74–78.

Ameling, J.M., Ephraim, P.L., Bone, L.R., Levine, D.M., Roter, D.L., Wolf, J.L., ... Hill-Briggs, F. (2014). Adapting hypertension self-management interventions to enhance their sustained effectiveness among urban African Americans. *Family & Community Health, 37*(2), 119–133.

American Heart Association. 2016. Coronary Artery Disease-Coronary Heart Disease. Accessed July 28, 2016. http://www.heart.org/HEARTORG/Conditions/More/MyHeartandStrokeNews/Coronary-Artery-Disease---Coronary-Heart-Disease_UCM_436416_Article.jsp#.V5kp9ZMrJmA.

American Heart Association Heart and Stroke Encyclopedia. 2016. Accessed July 10, 2016. http://www.heart.org/HEARTORG/Encyclopedia/Heart-Encyclopedia_UCM_445084_Encyclopedia.jsp?levelSelected=20&title=prehypertension.

Appel, L.J., Wright, J.T., Jr., Greene, T., Lawrence, Y., Agodoa, B.C., Astor, G.L., ... Bakris. (2010). Intensive blood-pressure control in hypertensive chronic kidney disease. *New England J Medicine, 363*(10), 918–929.

Arena, S.K., Drouin, J., Thompson, K.A., Black, R.E., & Peterson, E.L. (2014). Prevalence of pre-hypertension and hypertension blood pressure readings among individuals managed by physical therapists in the home care setting: A descriptive study. *Cardiopulmonary Physical Therapy J, 25*(1), 18–22.

Arslanian-Engoren, C. (2011). Women's risk factors and screening for coronary heart disease. *J Obstet Gynecol Neonatal Nursing, 40*(3), 337–347.

Azancot, M.A., Ramos, N., Moreso, F.J., Ibernon, M., Espinel, E., Torres, I.B., ... Seron, D.

(2014). Hypertension in chronic kidney disease: The influence of renal transplantation. *Transplantation, 98*(5), 537–542.

Azzi, M., Perdrix, L., Bobrie, G., Frank, M., Chatellier, G., Menard, J., & Plouin, P.F. (2014). Greater efficacy of aldosterone blockade and diuretic reinforcement vs. dual renin-angiotensin blockade for left ventricular mass regression in patients with resistant hypertension. *J Hypertension, 32*(10), 2038–2044.

Barksdale, D.J., & Metiko, E. (2010). The role of parental history of hypertension in predicting hypertension risk factors in black Americans. *J Transcultural Nursing, 21*(4), 306–313.

Bell, E.J., Lutsey, P.L., Windham, B.G., & Folsom, A.R. (2013). Physical activity and cardiovascular disease in African Americans in ARIC. *Med Sci Sports Exerc, 45*(5), 901–907.

Bennett, J. (2013). Beliefs and attitudes about medication adherence in African American men with high blood pressure. *MedSurg Matters Newsletter, 22*(3), 4–10.

Bier, D.M., Derelian, D., German, J.B., Katz, D.J., Pate, R.R., & Thompson, K.M. (2008). Improving compliance with dietary recommendations: Time for new, inventive approaches? *Nutrition Today, 43*(5), 180–187.

Boosman, H., Schepers, V.P.N., Post, M.M.M., & Viesser-Meily, J.M.A. (2011). Social activity contributes independently to life satisfaction three years post stroke. *Clinical Rehabilitation, 25,* 460–467.

Bosworth, H.B., Powers, B.J., Olsen, M.K., McCant, F., Grubber, J., Smith, V., ... Oddone, E.Z. (2011). Home blood pressure management and improved blood pressure control: Results from a randomized controlled trial. *Arch Intern Med, 171*(13), 1173–1180. DOI: 10.1001/archinternmed.2011.276.

Braunstein, J.B., Sherber, N.S., Schulman, S.P., Ding, E.L., & Powe, N.R. (2008). Race, medical researcher distrust, perceived harm, and willingness to participate in cardiovascular prevention trials. *Medicine, 87*(1), 1–9.

Bruce, M.A., Beech, B.M., Sims, M., Griffith, D.M., Simpson, S.L., Ard, J., & Norris, K.C. (2013). Sex, weight status, and chronic kidney disease among African Americans: The Jackson Heart Study. *J Investigative Medicine, 61*(4), 701–706.

Brunborg, B., & Ytrehus, S. (2013). Sense of well-being 10-years after stroke. *J Clinical Nursing, 23,* 1055–1063. DOI:10.1111/jocn.12324.

Bunker, J. (2014). Hypertension: Diagnosis, assessment and management. Nursing Standard, 28(42), 50–59.

Burla, M., Brody, A.M., Ference, B.A., Flack, J.M., Mahn, J.J., Marinica, A.L., ... Levy, P.D. (2014). Blood pressure control and perceived health status in African Americans with subclinical hypertensive heart disease. *J American Society of Hypertension, 8*(5), 321–329.

Cahill, L.E., Chiuve, S.E., Mekary, R.A., Jensen, M.K., Flint, A.J., Hu, F.B., & Rimm, E.B. (2013). Epidemiology and prevention: Prospective study of breakfast eating and incident coronary heart disease in a cohort of male U.S. health professionals. *Circulation, 128,* 313–314. D0I:10.1161/CIR.0b013e3182a366b7.

Cancarini, G. (2004). Long-term outcome in PD morbidity and mortality. *J Nephrol, 17,* S67-S71.

Canzanello, V.J., Baranco-Pryor, E., Rahbari-Oskoui, F., Schwartz, G.L., Boerwinkle, E., Turner, S.T., & Chapman, A.B. (2008). Predictors of blood pressure response to the angiotensin receptor blocker candesartan in essential hypertension. *American J Hypertension, 21*(1), 61–66.

Cardarelli, R., Cardarelli, K.M., Fulda, K.G., Espinoza, A., Cage, C., Vishwanatha, J., ... Carrol, J. (2010). Self-reported racial discrimination, response to unfair treatment, and coronary calcification in asymptomatic adults: The North Texas Healthy Heart Study. *BMC Public Health, 10,* 285.

Centers for Disease Control and Prevention [CDC]. (2011). Prevalence of coronary heart disease: United States 2006–2010. *J American Medical Association, 306*(19), 2084–2086.

Centers for Disease Control and Prevention [CDC]. (2012). High blood pressures facts. Retrieved March 29, 2012. http://www.cdc.gov/bloodpressure/facts.htm.

Centers for Disease Control and Prevention [CDC]. (2013.) Hypertension Among Adults in the United States: National Health and Nutrition Examination Survery, 2011–2012. NBGS Data Brief No. 133, Oct. 2013. Accessed July 12, 2016. http:www.cdc.gov/nchs/data/databriefs/db133.htm.

Centers for Disease Control and Prevention [CDC]. (2015.) High Blood Pressure Facts. Accessed July 12, 2016. http://www.cdc.gov/bloodpressure/facts.htm.

Chalmers, J., Arima, H., Harrap, S., Touyz, R.M., & Park, J.B. (2013). Global survey of current practice in management of hypertension as reported by societies affiliated with the International Society of Hypertension. *J Hypertension, 31*(5), 1043–1048.

Chapman, A.B., Schwartz, G.L., Boerwinkle, E., & Turner, S.T. (2002). Predictors of antihypertensive response to a standard dose of hydrochlorothiazide for essential hypertension. *Kidney International, 61*(3), 1047–1055.

Cheng, S., Gupta, D.K., Claggett, B., Sharrett, A.R., Shah, A.M., Skali, H., & Solomon, S.D. (2013). Differential influence of distinct components of increased blood pressure on cardiovascular outcomes: From the atherosclerosis risk in communities study. *Hypertension, 62*(3), 492–498. DOI:10.1161/Hypertensionaha.113.01561.

Chiha, M., Njeim, M., & Chedrawy, E.G. (2012). Diabetes and coronary heart disease: A risk factor for the global epidemic. *International J Hypertension*, 697240. DOI:10.1155/2012/697240.

Chiu, M., Austin, P.C., Manuel, D.G., & Tu, J.V. (2010). Comparison of cardiovascular risk profiles among ethnic groups using population health surveys between 1996 and 2007. *Canadian Medical Association J, 182*(8), e301–e310.

Chobanian, A.V. (2001). Control of hypertension: An important national priority. *New England J Medicine, 345*, 534–535. DOI:10.1056/NEJM200108163450709.

Chrysant, S.G., Littlejohn, T., III, Izzo J.L., Jr., Kereiakes, D.J., Oparil, S., Melino, M., ... Heyrman, R. (2012). Triple-combination therapy with olmesartan, amlodipine, and hydrochlorothiazide in black and non-black study participants with hypertension: The TRINITY randomized, double-blind, 12-week, parallel-group study. *AMJ Cardiovascular Drugs, 12*(4), 233–243.

Coly, G., Kotchen, J.M., Grim, C.E., Yang, H., Ow, A.J., Krishnaswami, S., & Kotchen, T.A. (2008). Characteristics of inner-city African Americans with uncontrolled hypertension. *J American Society of Hypertension, 2*(5), 366–371. DOI:10.1016/j.jash.2008.04.003.

Cooper, L.A., Roter, D.L., Carson, K.A., Bone, L.R., Larson, S.M., Miller, E.R., III, ... Levine, D.M. (2011). A randomized trial to improve patient-centered care and hypertension control in underserved primary care patients. *J Gen Intern Med, 26*(11), 1297–1304.

Cozier, Y., Palmer J.R., Horton, N.J., Fredman, L., Wise, L.A., & Rosenberg, L. (2006). Racial discrimination and the incidence of hypertension in U.S. black women. *Ann Epidemiol, 16*(9), 681–687. DOI:10.1016/j.annepidemi.2005.11.008.

Crowley, M.J., Powers, B.J., Olsen, M.K., Grubber, J.M., Koropchak, C., Rose, C.M., ... Bosworth, H.B. (2013). Diabetes and metabolism: The cholesterol, hypertension, and glucose education (CHANGE) study: Results from a randomized controlled trial in African Americans with diabetes. *American Heart J, 166*(1), 179–186.

Cuffee, Y.L., Hargraves, J.L., Rosal, M., Briesacher, B.A., Schoenthaler, A., Person, S., ... Allison, J. (2013). Reported racial discrimination, trust in physicians and medication adherence among inner-city African Americans with hypertension. *American J Public Health, 103*(11), e55–e62.

Daniels, L.B., Grady, D., Mosca, L., Collins, P., Mitlak, B., Amewou-Atisso, M., ... Barrett-Connor, E. (2013). Is diabetes mellitus a heart disease equivalent in women? Results from an international study of postmenopausal women in the raloxifene use for the heart

(RUTH) trial. *Circ Cardiovasc Qual Outcomes, 6*(2), 164–170. DOI:10.1161/Circoutcomes.112.966986.

De Caterina, A.R., and A.M. Leone. 2010. Why beta-blockers should not be used as a first choice in uncomplicated hypertension. *American Journal of Cardiology.* May 15;105(10):1433–8.

DeVore, A.D., Sorrentino, M., Arnsdorf, M.F., Ward, P., Bakris, G.L., & Blankstein, R. (2010). Predictors of hypertension control in a diverse general cardiology practice. *J Clinical Hypertension, 12*(8), 570–577.

Dodani, S. (2011). Community-based participatory research approaches for hypertension control and prevention in churches. *Int J Hypertension,* 273120. DOI:10.4061/2011/273120.

Drezner, M., Rosen, C., and J. Mulder. 2016. Patient information: Vitamin D deficiency (Beyond the Basics). *Up to Date.* Accessed Aug 2, 2016. http://www.uptodate.com/contents/vitamin-d-deficiency-beyond-the-basics.

Dusek, J.A., Hibberd, P.L., Buczynski, B., Chang, B.-H., Dusek, K.C., Johnston, J.M., ... Zusman, R.M. (2008). Stress management versus lifestyle modification on systolic hypertension and medication elimination: A randomized trial. *J Alternative Complementary Med, 14*(2), 129–138.

Eames, S., Hoffmann, T.C., & Phillips, N.F. (2014). Evaluating stroke patients' awareness of risk factors and readiness to change stroke risk-related behaviors in a randomized controlled trial. *Topics in Stroke Rehabilitation, 21 Suppl 1,* S52–S62.

Egan, B.M., and F. Stevens. 2015. Prehypertension-prevalence, health risks, and management strategies. Nature Reviews, Cardiology. May, 12: 289–300. Accessed July 10, 2016. http://www.nature.com/nrcardio/journal/v12/n5/full/nrcardio.2015.17.html.

Egan, B.M., Zhao, Y., Li, J., Brzezinski, A.W., Todoran, T.M., Brook, R.D., & Calhoun, T.M. (2013). Prevalence of optimal treatment regimens in patients with apparent treatment-resistant hypertension based on office blood pressure in a community-based practice network. *Hypertension, 62*(4), 691–697. DOI:10.1161/HypertensionAHA.113.01448.

Elder, K., Ramamonjiarivelo, Z., Wiltshire, J., Piper, C., Horn, W.S., Gilbert, K.L., ... Allison, J. (2012). Trust, medication adherence, and hypertension control in southern African American men. *American J Public Health, 102*(12), 2242–2245.

Erem, C., Hacihasanoglu, A., Kocak, M., Deger, O., & Topbas, M. (2008). Prevalence of prehypertension and hypertension and associated risk factors among Turkish adults: Trabzon Hypertension Study. *J Public Health, 31*(1), 47–58. DOI:10.1093/pubmed/fdn078.

Falcone, G.J., Biffi, A., Devan, W.J., Jagiella, J.M., Schmidt, H., Kissela, B., ... Rosand, J. (2012). Burden of risk alleles for hypertension increases risk of intracerebral hemorrhage. *Stroke,* 43(11), 2877–2883. DOI:10.1161/Strokeaha.112.659755.

Fan, A.Z., Stephnie, D., Mallawaarachchi, V., Gilbertz, D., Li, Y., & Mokdad, A.H. (2010). Lifestyle behaviors and receipt of preventive health care services among hypertensive Americans aged 45 years or older in 2007. *Preventive Medicine, 50,* 138–142.

Farley, H.F., & Miller, P.L. (1987). Assessment of the urinary function. In W.J. Phipps, B.C. Long, & N.F. Woods (Eds.), *Medical-Surgical Nursing: Concepts and Clinical Practice,* 3rd edition (pp. 1577–1593). St. Louis: Mosby.

Feng, X.L., Pang, M., & Beard, J. (2014). Health system strengthening and hypertension awareness, treatment and control: Data from the China health and retirement longitudinal study. *Bull World Organ, 92,* 29–41. DOI:10.2471/BLT.13.124495.

Ferdinand, K.C., Pool, J., Weitzman, R., Purkayastha, D., & Townsend, R. (2011). Peripheral and central blood pressure responses of combination aliskiren/hydrochlorothiazide and amlodipine monotherapy in African American patients with Stage 2 hypertension: The ATLAAST trial. *J Clinical Hypertension, 13*(5), 366–375.

Ferdinand, K.C., & Townsend, R.R. (2012). Hypertension in the U.S. black population: Risk factors, complications, and potential impact of central aortic pressure on effective treatment. *Cardiovascular Drugs Therapy, 26,* 157–165.

Fernandez, S., Tobin, J.N., Cassells, A., Diaz-Gloster, M., Kalida, C., & Ogedegbe, G. (2011). The counseling African Americans to control hypertension (CAATCH) trial: Baseline demographic, clinical, psychosocial, and behavioral characteristics. *Implementation Science, 6*(100), 1–13.

Fiscella, K., & Franks, P. (2010). Vitamin D, race and cardiovascular mortality: Findings from a national U.S. sample. *Annals of Family Medicine, 8,* 11–18.

Fiscella, K., Winters, P., Tancredi, D., & Franks, P. (2011). Racial disparity in blood pressure: Is vitamin D a factor? *J Gen Intern Med, 26*(10), 1105–1111.

Flack, J.M., Sica, D.A., Bakris, G., Brown, A.L., Ferdinand, K.C., Grimm Jr., R.H., ... Jamerson, K.A. (2010). Management of high blood pressure in blacks: An update of the International Society on Hypertension in blacks consensus statement. *Hypertension, 56*(5), 780–800. DOI:10.1161/HypertensionAHA.110.152892.

Fogoros, R.N. (2011). *Prehypertension.* Retrieved September 19, 2013, from http://heartdisease.about.com/od/highbloodpressure/a/Prehypertension.htm.

Folson, A.R., Parker, E.D., & Harnack, L.J. (2007). Degree of concordance with DASH diet guidelines and incidence of hypertension and fatal cardiovascular disease. *American J Hypertension, 20,* 225–232. DOI:10.1016/j.amjhyper.2006.09.003.

Frankenfield, D.L., Rocco, M.V., Roman, S.H., & McClellan, W.M. (2003). Survival advantage for adult Hispanic hemodialysis patients? Findings from the end stage renal disease clinical performance measures project. *American Society of Nephrology, 12,* 180–186.

Freedman, B.I., Wagenknecht, L.E., Hairston, K.G., Bowden, D.W., Carr, J.J., Hightower, R.C., ... Divers, J. (2010). Vitamin D, adiposity, and calcified atherosclerotic plaque in African-Americans. *J Clinical Endocrinology & Metabolism, 95*(3), 1076–1083.

Gallagher, B.D., Muntner, P. Moise, N., Lin, J.J., & Kronish, I.M. (2015). Are two commonly used self-report questionnaires useful for identifying antihypertensive medication non-adherence? *J Hypertension,* 33(1), 1–6.

Gaziano, T.A., Bitton, A., Anand, S., Abrahams-Gessel, & Murphy, A. (2010). Growing epidemic of coronary heart disease in low and middle-income countries. *Curr Probl Cardiol,* 35(2), 72–115.

Gill, J.S., Rose, C., Pereira, B.J.G., & Tonelli, M. (2007). The importance of transitions between dialysis and transplantation in the care of end-stage renal disease patients. *Kidney International, 71*(5), 442–447.

Ginde, A.A., Scragg, R., Schwartz, R.S., & Camargo, C.A. (2009). Prospective study of serum 25-hydroxyvitamin D level, cardiovascular disease mortality, and all-cause mortality in older U.S. adults. *J Am Geriatric Soc, 57*(9), 1595–1603.

Go, A.S., Mozaffarian, D., Roger, V.L., Benjamin, E.J., Berry, J.D., Blaha, M.J. ... Turner, M.B. (2014). AHA statistical update. Executive summary: Heart disease and stroke statistics—2014 update. A report from the American Heart Association. *Circulation, 129,* 399–410. DOI:10.1161/01.cir.0000442015.53336.12.

Goldman, Lee. 2015. *Too Much of a Good Thing: How Four Key Survival Traits Are Now Killing Us.* New York: Little, Brown, and Company.

Gross, B., Anderson, E.F., Busby, S., Frith, K.H., & Panco, C.E. (2013). Using culturally sensitive education to improve adherence with anti-hypertension regimen. *J Cultural Diversity, 20*(2), 75–79.

Gu, D., Zhao, Q., Chen, J., Chen, J.-C., Huang, J., Bazzano, L.A. ... He, J. (2013). Reproducibility of blood pressure responses to dietary sodium and potassium interventions: The GenSalt study. *Hypertension, 62*(3), 499–505. DOI:10.1161/HYPERTENSIONAHA.113.01034.

Gutierrez, J., & Williams, O.A. (2014). Global Perspectives. *Neurology, 82,* 1080–1082.

Hageman, P.A., Carol, H., Pullen, S., Noble, W., & Boeckner, L. (2010). Blood pressure, fitness, and lipid profiles of rural women in the Wellness for Women project. *Cardiopulmonary Physical Therapy J, 21*(3), 27–34.

Harjutsalo, V., & Groop, P.H. (2014). Epidemiology and risk factors for diabetic kidney disease. *Advances in Chronic Kidney Disease, 21*(3), 260–266.

Harris, S.S. (2006). Symposium optimizing vitamin D intake for populations with special needs: Barriers to effective food fortification and supplementation. *J Nutrition, 136*(4), 1126–1129.

______. (2011). Does vitamin D deficiency contribute to increased rates of cardiovascular disease and type 2 diabetes in African Americans? *Am J Clin Nutr, 93*(5), 1175S–8S.

Hatori, N., Sakai, H., Sato, K., Mitani, K., Miyajima, M., Yuasa, S., ... Miyakawa, M. (2014). Changes in blood-pressure control among patients with hypertension from 2008 through 2011: Surveys of actual clinical practice. *J Nippon Medical School, 81* (4), 258–263.

Heart and Stroke Foundation of Canada. (2014a). *Stroke: What Is a Stroke?* Retrieved December 1, 2014, from http://www.heartandstroke.com/site/c.ikIQLcMWJtE/b.3483935/k.736A/Stroke_What_is_Stroke.htm.

Heart and Stroke Foundation of Canada. (2014b). *Stroke: Stroke Signs.* Retrieved December 1, 2014, from http://www.heartandstroke.com/site/c.ikIQLcMWJtE/b.3483937/k.86D8/Stroke_Stroke_signs.htm.

Hernandez-Villa, Eduardo. (2015). A Review of the JNC 8 Blood Pressure Guideline. *Texas Heart Institute Journal.* Jun; 42(3): 226–8.

Hicken, M.T., Lee, H., Morenoff, J., House, J.S., & Williams, D.R. (2014). Racial/ethnic disparities in hypertension prevalence: Reconsidering the role of chronic stress. *American J Public Health, 104*(1), 117–123.

High blood pressure risk factors. (2013, June 27). *New York Times.* http://health.nytimes.com/health/guides/disease/hypertension/risk-factor.html.

Holt, E., Joyce, C., Dornelles, A., Morisky, D., Webber, L.S., Muntner, P., & Krousel-Wood, M. (2013). Sex differences in barriers to antihypertensive medication adherence: Findings from the cohort study of medication adherence among older adults. *J Am Geriatric Soc, 61*(4), 558–564.

Horigan, A., Rocciccioli, J., & Trimm, D. (2012). Dialysis and fatigue: Implications for nurses—A case study analysis. *Medsurg Nursing, 21*(3), 158–175.

Houston, M. (2011). The role of magnesium in hypertension and cardiovascular disease. *J Clinical Hypertension, 13*(11), 843–847.

Howard, D.L., Carson, A.P., Holmes, D.N., & Kaufman, J.S. (2009). Consistency of care and blood pressure control among elderly African Americans and whites with hypertension. *J Am Board Fam Med, 22*(3), 307–315. DOI:10.3122/jabfm.2009.03.080145.

Howard, G., Lackland, D.T., Kleindorfer, D.O., Kissela, B.M., Moy, C.S., Judd, S., ... Howard, V.J. (2013). Racial differences in the impact of elevated systolic blood pressure on stroke. *JAMA Intern Med, 173*(1), 46–51. DOI:10.1001/2013.jamainternmed.857.

Hunt, S.A., Abraham, W.T., Chin, M.H., Feldman, A.M., Francis, G.S., Ganiats, T.G., ... Yancy, C.W. (2005). ACC/AHA practice guidelines: ACC/AHA 2005 guideline update for the diagnosis and management of chronic heart failure in the adult. *Circulation, 112,* 1825–1852. DOI:10.1161/CirculationAHA.105.167587.

Ibrahim, H.N., Wang, C., Ishani, A., Collins, A.J., & Foley, R.N. (2008). Screening for chronic kidney disease complications in U.S. adults: Racial implications of a single GFR threshold. *Clinical J American Society of Nephrology, 3,* 1792–1799.

Inker, L.A., Coresh, J., Levey, A.S., Tonelli, M., & Muntner, P. (2011).Estimated GFR, albuminuria, and complications of chronic kidney disease. *J Am Soc Nephrol, 22*(12), 2322–2331. DOI:10.1681/ASN.2010111181.

James, M.T., Hemmelgarn, B.R., & Tonelli, M. (2010). Early recognition and prevention of chronic kidney disease. *Lancet, 375*(9722), 1296–1309. DOI:10.1016/S0140-6736(09)62004-3. [Erratum in *Lancet, 376*(9736):162.]

James, P., Oparil, S., Carter, B., Cushman, W., Dennison-Himmelfarb, C., Handler, J., Lackland, D., LeFevre, M., MacKenzie, T., Ogedegbe, O., Smith, S., Svetkley, L., Tater, S., Townsend,

R., Wright, J., Narva, A., and Eduardo Ortiz. 2014. Evidence-Based Guideline for the Management of High Blood Pressure in Adults: Report From the Panel Members Appointed to the Eighth Joint National Committee (JNC 8). *Journal of the American Medical Association*. 311(5): 507–20.

Jayasekara, R. (2009). The psychosocial spiritual experience of elderly individuals recovering from stroke: A systematic review. *J Advanced Nursing, 65*(5), 965–970.

Joffres, M., Falaschetti, E., Gillespite, C., Robitaille, C., Loustalot, F., Poulter, N., McAlister, F., Johansen, J., Baclic, O., and N. Campbell. 2013. Hypertension prevalence, awareness, treatment and control in national surveys from England, the USA and Canada, and correlation with stroke and ischaemic heart disease mortality: a cross-sectional study. *British Medical Journal Open*, August. Accessed July 19, 2016. http://bmjopen.bmj.com/content/3/8/e003423.full.

Jorgensen, R.S., & Maisto, S.A. (2008). Alcohol consumption and prehypertension: An investigation of university youth. *Behavioral Medicine, 34*, 21–26.

Judd, S.E., Nanes, M.S., Ziegler, T. R., Wilson, P.W.F., & Tangpricha, V. (2008). Optimal vitamin D status attenuates the age-associated increase in systolic blood pressure in white Americans: Results from the third National Health and Nutrition Examination Survey. *American J Clinical Nutrition, 87*, 136–141.

Judd, S.E., Raiser, S.N., Kumari, M., & Tangpricha, V. (2010). 1,25-Dihydroxyvitamin D_3 reduces systolic blood pressure in hypertensive adults: A pilot feasibility study. *J Steroid Biochemistry Molecular Biology, 121*, 445–447.

Kalache, G. 2015. High Blood Pressure: Hypertension could be autoimmune disease, study finds. *News, The World Today*, Sept. 9: 1–2.

Kaplan, N.M., & Lieberman, E. (1998). *Clinical Hypertension*, 7th edition. Baltimore: Williams & Wilkins.

Karpinos, A.R., Roumie, C.L., Nian, H., Diamond, A.B., & Rothman, R.L. (2013). High prevalence of hypertension among collegiate football athletes. *Cardiovasc Qual Outcomes, 6*, 716–723. DOI:10.1161/Circoutcomes.113.000463.

Kavanagh, J.M. (1987). Assessment of the cardiovascular system. In W.J. Phipps, B.C. Long, & N.F. Woods (Eds.), *Medical-Surgical Nursing: Concepts and Clinical Practice*, 3rd edition. St. Louis: Mosby.

Kearne, P., Whelton, M., Reynolds, K., Muntner, P., Whelton, P., and He Jiang. 2005. Global burden of hypertension: analysis of worldwide data. *The Lancet*, Jan (365): 217–23.

Kem, D., Yu, X., Patterson, E., Huang, S., Stavrakis, S., Szabo, B., Olansky, L., McCauley, J., and M.W. Cunningham. 2007. Hypertension Case Report: Autoimmune Hypertensive Syndrome. *Hypertension*; 50: 829–34.

Kent, S.T., Shimbo, D., Huang, L., Diaz, K.M., Kilgore, M.L., Oparil, S., & Muntner, P. (2014). Antihypertensive medication classes used among Medicare beneficiaries initiating treatment in 2007–2010. *PLoS ONE, 9*(8), e105888. DOI:10.1371/journal.pone.0105888.

Khalil, A.A., Darawad, M., Gamal, E.A.L., Hamdan-Mansour, A.M., & Abed, M.A. (2012). Predictors of dietary and fluid non-adherence in Jordanian patients with end-stage renal disease receiving hemodialysis: A cross-sectional study. *J Clinical Nursing, 22*, 127–136.

Khara, K. (2010). *Function of vitamin D*. http://www.buzzle.com/articles/function-of-vitamin-d.html.

Khare, M.M., Huber, R., Carpenter, R.A., Balmer, P.W., Bates, N.J., Nolen, K.N., ... Will, J.C. (2009). A lifestyle approach to reducing cardiovascular risk factors in undeserved women: Design and methods of the Illinois WISEWOMAN Program. *J Women's Health, 18*(3), 409–419.

Kidney Foundation of Canada. (2010). *Some facts about central venous catheters (hemodialysis catheters)*. Retrieved April 19, 2014, from http://www.kidney.ca/document.doc?id-764.

Kidney Foundation of Canada. (2014). *Peritoneal dialysis*. Retrieved April 19, 2014, from http://www.kidney.ca/peritoneal-dialysis.

Kolasa, K.M., Sollid, K., Smith Edge, M., & Bouchoux, A. (2012). Blood pressure management: Communicating comprehensive lifestyle strategies beyond sodium. *Nutrition Today, 47*(4), 183–190.

Koliaki C., & Katsilambros, N. (2013). Dietary sodium, potassium, and alcohol: Key players in the pathophysiology, prevention, and treatment of human hypertension. *Nutrition in Clinical Care: Nutrition Reviews, 71*(6), 402–411.

Konerman, M., Weeks, K.R., Shands, J.R., Tiburt, J.C., Dy, S., Bone, L.R., Levine, D.M., & Young, J.H. (2011). Short Form (SF-36) Health Survey measures are associated with decreased adherence among urban African Americans with severe, poorly controlled hypertension. *J Clinical Hypertension, 13*(5), 385–390.

Krakoff, L.R. (2011). Management of cardiovascular risk factors is leaving the office: Potential impact of telemedicine. *J Clinical Hypertension, 13*(11), 791–794.

Kramer, A.B., van der Meulen, E.F., Hamming, I., van Goor, H., & Navis, G. (2007). Effect of combining ACE inhibition with aldosterone blockade on proteinuria and renal damage in experimental nephrosis. *International Society of Nephrology, 71*(5), 417–424.

Kugler, Mary. 2016. Autoimmune Kidney Disease, IgA Nephropathy. *Very Well Health*. March 28. Accessed Aug 4, 2016. https://www.verywell.com/autoimmune-kidney-disease-286 0360

Lakshminarayan, K., Berger, A.K., Fuller, C.C., Jacobs Jr., D.R., Anderson, D.C., Steffen, L.M., ... Luepker, R.V. (2014). Trends in 10-year survival of patients with stroke hospitalized between 1980 and 2000: The Minnesota stroke survey. *Stroke, 45*(9), 2575–2581. DOI:10.1161/Strokeaha.114.005512.

Lameire, N., & Biesen, W.V. (2004). Hypervolemia in peritoneal dialysis patients. *J Nephrology, 17*(suppl 8), S58–S66.

Lavie, C.J., DiNicolantonio, J.J., Milani, R.V., & O'Keefe, J.H. (2013). Vitamin D and cardiovascular health. *Circulation, 128*, 2404–2406. DOI:10.1161/Circulation AHA.113.002 902.

Lefler, L.L., & Nuss, R.L. (2009). Double Jeopardy! Heart disease risk factors for older African American and Caucasian women. *Medsurgical Nursing, 18*(6), 347–354.

Leung, L.B., Busch, A.M., Nottage, S.L., Arellano, N., Glieberman, E., Busch, N.J., & Smith, S.R. (2012). Approach to antihypertensive adherence: A feasibility study on the use of student health coaches for uninsured hypertensive adults. *Behavioral Medicine, 38*, 19–27.

Lewis, L.M., Askie, P., Randleman, S., & Shelton-Dunston, B. (2010). Medication adherence beliefs of community-dwelling hypertensive African Americans. *J Cardiovascular Nursing, 25*(3), 199–206.

Li, W.W, Kuo, C.T., Hwang, S.L., & Hsu, H.T. (2012). Factors related to medication nonadherence for patients with hypertension in Taiwan. *J Clinical Nursing, 21*, 1816–1824. DOI:10.1111/j1365-2702.2012.04008.x.

Liu, M., Li, Y., Wei, F., Zhang, L., Han, J., & Wang, J. (2013). Is high blood pressure load associated, independently of blood pressure level, with target organ damage? *J Hypertension, 31*(9), 1812–1818.

Lok, C.E., & Foley, R. (2013). Vascular access morbidity and mortality: Trends of the last decade. *Clin J Am Nephrol, 8*, 1213–1219.

Lunardo, Emily. 2016. Blood Pressure 2016: updated measurement guidelines generate controversy even as hypertension cases rise. Bel Marra Health. Accessed July 10, 2016. http://www.belmarrahealth.com/category/blood-pressure.

Ma, C., Chen, S., You, L., Luo, Z., & Xing, C. (2011). Development and psychometric evaluation of the treatment adherence questionnaire for patients with hypertension. *J Advanced Nursing, 68*(6), 1402-1413. DOI:10.1111/j.1365-2648.2011.05835.x.

MacKenzie, G., Ireland, S., Moore, S., Heinz, I., Johnson, R., Oczkowski, W., & Sahlas, D. (2013). Tailored interventions to improve hypertension management after stroke or TIA-phase II (TIMS II). *Canadian J Neuroscience Nursing, 35*(1), 27–34.

Madhur, M., and Maron, D. 2014. Hypertension Treatment & Management. *Medscape*. September 30.

Madhur, M.S., Riaz, K.R., Dreisbach, A.W., & Harrison, D.G. (2014). *Hypertension*. Maron, D.J. (Ed.). Retrieved July 6, 2015, from http://emedicine.medscape.com/article/241381.

Magid, D.J., Olson, K.L., Billups, S.J., Wagner, N.M., Lyons, E.E., & Kroner, B.A. (2013). A pharmacist-led American Heart Association Heart 360 web-enabled home blood pressure monitoring program. *Circ Cardovasc Qual Outcomes, 6*, 157–163. DOI:10.1161/Circoutcomes.112.968172.

Manze, M., Rose, A.J., Orner, M.B., Berlowitz, D.R., & Kressin, N.R. (2010). Understanding racial disparities in treatment intensification for hypertension management. *J Gen Intern Med, 25*(8), 819–825. DOI:10.1007/s11606-010-1342-9.

Martins, D., Agodoa, L., & Norris, K.C. (2012). Hypertensive chronic kidney disease in African Americans: Strategies for improving care. *Cleveland Clinical J Med, 79*(10), 1–14.

Mayo Clinic. Prehypertension Risk Factors. 2015, June 23. Accessed July 11, 2016. http://www.mayoclinic.org/diseases-conditions/prehypertension/basics/risk-factors/con-200 26271.

McCauley, K.M. (2007). Modifying women's risk for cardiovascular disease. *J Obstet Gynecol Neonatal Nursing, 36*(2), 116–124.

McDonnell, M.N., Hillier, S.L., Hooker, S.P., Le, A., Judd, S.E., & Howard, V.J. (2013). Physical activity frequency and risk of incident stroke in a national U.S. study of blacks and whites. *Stroke, 44*, 2519–2524. DOI:10.1161/Strokeaha.113.001538.

Melamed, M.L., Astor, B., Michos, E.D., Hostetter, T.H., & Powe, N.R. (2009). 25-hydroxyvitamin D levels, race, and the progression of kidney disease. *J American Society Nephrology, 20*, 2631–2639.

Millasseau, S., Kelly, R., Ritter, J., and P. Chowiencyzy. 2002. Determination of age-related increases in large artery stiffness by digital pulse contour analysis. *Clinical Science*, 103: 371–7.

Mitka, M. (2011). Lifestyle changes key to cut stroke risk. Guidelines place emergency physicians on front line. *J American Medical Association, 305*(6), 551–552.

Moe, G.W., & Tu, J. (2010). Heart failure in the ethnic minorities. *Curr Opin Cardiol, 25*,124–130. DOI:101097/NCO.0b013e328335fea4.

Moore, D.R., Feurer, I.D., Zaydfudim, V., Hoy, H., Zavala, E.Y., Shaffer, D., ... Moore, D.E. (2012). Evaluation of living kidney donors: Variables that affect donation. *Progress in Transplantation, 22*(4), 385–392.

Moore, T.J., Karanja, N., Svetkey, L.P., & Jenkins, M. (2011). Why DASH? Hypertension: The silent killer. In T.J. Moore (Ed.), *The DASH Diet for Hypertension: Lower your Blood Pressure in 14 Days—Without Drugs* (pp. 11–19). New York: Gallery Books.

Morbidity and Mortality Weekly Report [MMWR]. (2009). Application of lower sodium intake recommendations to adults—United States, 1999–2006. *Weekly, 58*(11); 281–283. http://www.cdc.gov/mmwr/preview/mmwrhtml/mm5811a2.htm.

Morbidity and Mortality Weekly Report [MMWR]. (2013). Vital signs: Avoidable deaths from heart disease, stroke, and hypertensive disease—United States, 2001–2010. *Weekly, 62*(35), 721–727. http://www.cdc.gov/mmwr/preview/mmwrhtml/mm6235a4.htm.

Motiwala, S.R., & Wang, T.J. (2011). Vitamin D and cardiovascular disease. *Curr Opin Nephrol Hypertension, 20*, 345–353. DOI:10.1097/MNH.0b013e3283474985.

Moyad, Mark. 2009. Vitamin D: A Rapid Review. *Dermatology Nursing*, 21(1); accessed Aug 1, 2016. http://www.medscape.com/viewarticle/589256_4

Munger, M.A. (2010). Polypharmacy and combination therapy in the management of hypertension in elderly patients with co-morbid diabetes mellitus. *Drugs Aging, 27*(11), 871–883.

National Institutes of Health (NIH). 2015. Landmark NIH study shows intensive blood pressure management may save lives. Sept 11 Press Release. Accessed July 12, 2016. https://

www.nih.gov/news-events/news-releases/landmark-nih-study-shows-intensive-blood-pressure-management-may-save-lives.

National Kidney and Urologic Diseases Information Clearinghouse. 2012. Kidney Disease Statistics for the United States. Accessed Aug 8, 2016. https://www.niddk.nih.gov/health-information/health-statistics/Documents/KU_Diseases_Stats_508.pdf.

National Kidney Foundation. (2006). *Hemodialysis: What you need to know.* https://www.kidney.org/sites/default/files/docs/hemodialysis.pdf.

National Kidney Foundation. (2014). *Fast Facts.* Retrieved March 6, 2014, from http://www.kidney.org/news/newsroom/factsheets/FastFacts.cfm.

Nead, K.T., Zhou, M.M., Caceres, R.D., Olin, J.W., Cooke, J.P., & Leeper, N.J. (2013). Walking impairment questionnaire improves mortality risk prediction models in a high-risk cohort independent of peripheral arterial disease status. *Cir Cardiovasc Qual Outcomes, 6,* 255–261. DOI:10.1161/Circoutcomes.111.000070.

Nesbitt, S., Shojaee, A., & Maa, J.F. (2014). Efficacy/safety of a fixed-dose amlodipine/olmesartan medoxomil-based treatment regimen in hypertensive blacks and non-blacks with uncontrolled blood pressure on prior antihypertensive monotherapy. *J Clinical Hypertension, 15*(4), 247–253.

Neville, J. (1987). Assessment of nutritional status and dietary counseling. W.J. Phipps, B.C. Long, & N.F. Woods (Eds.), *Medical-Surgical Nursing: Concepts and Clinical Practice,* 3rd edition (pp. 1421–1449). St. Louis: Mosby.

Nogueira, J.M., Weir, M.R., Jacobs, S., Haririan, A., Breault, D., Klassen, D., … Cooper, M. (2009). A study of renal outcomes in African American living kidney donors. *Transplantation, 88*(12), 1371–1376. DOI:10.1097/TP.0b013e3.

Norris, K.C., Tareen, N., Martins, D., & Vaziri, N.D. (2008). Implications of ethnicity for the treatment of hypertensive kidney disease, with an emphasis on African Americans. *Nature Clinical Practice Nephrology, 4*(10), 538–549.

Nunes, J.A.W., Wallston, K.A., Eden, S.K., Shintani, A.K., Ikizler, T.A., & Cavanaugh, K.L. (2011). Associations among perceived and objective disease knowledge and satisfaction with physician communication in patients with chronic kidney disease. *Kidney International, 80*(12), 1344–1351.

O'Brien, E., Parati, G., & Stergiou, G. (2013). Ambulatory blood pressure measurement: What is the international consensus? *Hypertension, 62,* 988–994.

O'Brien, S.R., Xue, Y., Ingersoll, G., & Kelly, A. (2013). Shorter length of stay is associated with worse functional outcomes for Medicare beneficiaries with stroke. *Physical Therapy, 93*(12), 1592–1602.

Ofili, E.O., Zappe, D.H., Purkayastha, D., Samuel, R., & Sowers, J.R. (2013). Antihypertensive and metabolic effects of angiotensin receptor blocker/diuretic combination therapy in obese, hypertensive African Amercan and white patients. *American J Therapeutics, 20*(1), 1–12.

Ohene-Frempong, K., Weiner, S., Sleeper, L., Miller, S., Embury, S., Moohr, J., Wethers, D., Pegelow, C., Gill, F., and the Cooperative Study of Sickle Cell Disease. 1998. Cerebrovascular Accidents in Sickle Cell Disease: Rates and Risk Factors. *Blood Journal,* Jan: 288–94.

O'Shea, R., & Goode, O.R. (2013). Effects of stroke on informal carers. *Nursing Standard, 28*(15), 43–47.

Ostchega, Y., Huges, J.P., Wright, J.D., McDowell, M.A., & Louis, T. (2008). Are demographic characteristics, health care access and utilization, and comorbid conditions associated with hypertension among U.S. adults? *American J Hypertension, 21*(2), 159–165.

Palmer-Thierry, M., Henderson, V.M., Hammali, R.E.L., Cephas, S., Placios, C., Martin, B.R., & Weaver, C.M. (2008). Black and white female adolescents lose vitamin D metabolites into urine. *American J Medical Sciences, 335*(4), 278–283.

Park, Y.-H., Chang, H., Kim, J., & Kwak, S. (2012). Patient-tailored self-management intervention for older adults with hypertension in a nursing home. *J Clinical Nursing, 22*, 710–722. DOI:10.1111/j.1365-2702.2012.04236.x.

Park, Y.-H., Kim, H., Jang, S.-N., & Koh, C.K. (2013). Predictors of adherence to medication in older Korean patients with hypertension. *European J Cardiovascular Nursing, 12*(1), 17–24.

Pasucci, M.A., Leasure, R., Belknap, D.C., & Kodumthara, E. (2010). Situational challenges that impact health adherence in vulnerable populations. *J Cultural Diversity: An Interdisciplinary J, 17*(1), 4–12.

Peralta, C.A., Katz, R., Newman, A.B., Psaty, B.M., & Odden, M.C. (2014). Systolic and diastolic blood pressure, incident cardiovascular events, and death in elderly persons: The role of functional limitation in the cardiovascular health study. *Hypertension, 64*(3), 472–80. DOI:10.1161HYPERTENSIONAHA.114.03831.

Peralta, C.A., Weekley, C.C., Li, Y., & Shlipak, M.G. (2013). Occult chronic kidney disease among persons with hypertension in the United States: Data from the national health and nutrition surveys 1988–1994 and 1999–2002. *J Hypertension, 31*(6), 1196–1202. DOI:10.1097/HJH.0b013e32836.

Perin, M.S., Cornelio, M.E., Rodrigues, R.C., & Gallani, M.C.B.J. (2013). Characterization of salt consumption among hypertensives according to socio-demographic and clinical factors. *Rev Latino-Am Enfermagem, 21*(5), 1013–1021.

Peters, R.M., Aroian, K.J., & Flack. J.M. (2006). African American culture and hypertension prevention. *West J Nurs Res, 28*(7), 831–863. DOI:101177/0193945906289332.

Peterson, G.E., de Backer, T., Contreras, G., Wang, X., Kendrick, C., Greene, T., ... Phillips, R.A. (2013). Relationship of left ventricular hypertrophy and diastolic function with cardiovascular and renal outcomes in African Americans with hypertensive chronic kidney disease. *Hypertension, 62*, 518–525. DOI:10.1161/hypertensionAHA.111.00904.

Pfeifer, M., Begerow, B., Minne, H.W., Nachtigall, D., and C. Hansen. (2009). Effects of a Short-Term Vitamin D3 and Calcium Supplementation on Blood Pressure and Parathyroid Hormone Levels in Elderly Women. Journal of Clinical Endocrinology and Metabolism. July. Accessed July 31, 2016. http://press.endocrine.org/doi/full/10.1210/jcem.86.4.7393.

Pilz, S., Tomaschitz, A., Marz, W., Drechsler, C., Ritz, E., Zittermann, A., ... Dekker, J.M. (2011). Vitamin D, cardiovascular disease and mortality. *Clinical Endocrinology, 75*, 575–584. DOI:10.1111/j.1365-2265.2011.04147x.

PL Detail-Document, Treatment of Hypertension: JNC 8 and More. *Pharmacist's Letter/Prescriber's Letter*. February 2014.

Pletcher, M.J., Bibbins-Domingo, K., Lewis, C.E., Wei, G.S., Sidney, S., Carr, J.J., ... Hulley, S.B. (2014). Prehypertension during young adulthood and coronary calcium later in life. *Annals of Internal Medicine, 149*(2), 91–99.

Pniewski, J., Chodakowska-Zebrowska, M., Wozniak, R., Stepien, K. & Stafiej, A. (2003). Plasma homocysteine level and the course of ischemic stroke. *Acta Neurobiol Exp (Wars)*, *63*(2), 127–130.

Powell-Wiley, T.M., Banks-Richard, K., Williams-King, E., Tong, L., Ayers, C.R., deLemos, J.A., ... DeHaven, M.J. (2012). Churches as targets for cardiovascular disease prevention: Comparison of genes, nutrition, exercise, wellness and spiritual growth (GoodNEWS) and Dallas County populations. *J Public Health, 35*(1), 99–106. DOI:10.1093/pubmed/fds060.

Preidt, Robert. 2015. Lupus Death Rates Vary by Race, Ethnicity: Study; Asians, Hispanics most likely to survive the autoimmune disease. WebMD Jan 15. Accessed Aug 4, 2016. http://www.webmd.com/lupus/news/20150115/lupus-death-rates-vary-by-race-ethnicity-study-finds

Qaseem, A., Hopkins, R.H., Sweet, D.E., Starkey, M., & Shekelle, P. (2013). Screening, monitoring, and treatment of stage 1–3 chronic kidney disease: A clinical guideline from the American College of Physician. *Annals of Internal Medicine, 159*(12), 835–847.

Quinones, A.R., Liang, J., & Ye, W. (2012). Racial and ethnic differences in hypertension risk: New diagnoses after age 50. *Ethnicity & Disease, 22*, 175–180.

Radhakrishnan, K. (2011). The efficacy of tailored interventions for self-management outcomes of type 2 diabetes, hypertension or heart disease: A systematic review. *J Advanced Nursing, 68*(3), 496–510.

Ram, C.V., Ramaswamy, K., Qian, C., Biskupiak, J., Ryan, A., Quah, R., & Russo, P.A. (2011). Blood pressure outcomes in patients receiving angiotensin II receptor blockers in primary care: A comparative effectiveness analysis from electronic medical record data. *J Clinical Hypertension, 13*(11), 801–812.

Riaz, K., Bataman, V., ... et al. (2011). Hypertension. Medscape Reference Drugs Diseases Procedures. Updated Aug. 10, 2011. Retrieved http://emedicine.medscape.com/article/241381-overview, 12/08/2014, p. 1–16.

Rigsby, B.D. (2011). Hypertension improvement through healthy lifestyle modifications. *ABNF Journal, 22*(2), 41–43.

Ritz, E. (2007). Hypertension: The kidney is the culprit even in the absence of kidney disease. *Kidney International*, 371–372. DOI:10.1038\sj.ki5002142.

Robbins, C.L., Keyserling, T., Pitts, S.B., Morrow, J., Majette, N., Sisneros, J.A., ... Dietz, P.M. (2013). Screening low-income women of reproductive age for cardiovascular disease risk factors. *J Women's Health, 22*(4), 314–321.

Robinson-Cohen, C., Hoofnagle, A.N., Ix, J.H., Sachs, M.C., Tracy, R.P., Siscovick, D.S., ... deBoer, I.H. (2013). Racial differences in the association of serum 25-hydroxyvitamin D concentration with coronary heart disease events. *J American Medical Association, 310*(2), 179–188.

Rosano, C., Longstreth, W.T., Jr., Boudreau, R., Taylor, C.A., Du, Y., Kuller, L.H., & Newman, A.B. (2011). High blood pressure accelerates gait slowing in well-functioning older adults over 18-years of follow-up. *J Am Geriatr Soc 59*(3), 390–397.

Rostand, S.G. (2010). Vitamin D, blood pressure, and African Americans: Toward a unifying hypothesis. *Clinical J American Society of Nephrology, 5*, 1697–1703. DOI:10.22215/CJN.02960410.

Sakamoto, R., Jaceldo-Siegl, K., Haddad, E., Oda, K., Fraser, G.E., & Tonstad, S. (2013). Relationship of vitamin D levels to blood pressure in a bi-ethnic population. *Nutrition Metabolism and Cardiovascular Disease, 23*, 776–784.

Sarafidis, P.A., Georgianos, P., and G.L. Bakris. (2013). Resistant hypertension—its identification and epidemiology. *Nature Reviews Nephrology*; Jan; 9(1): 51–8.

Schneider, A.L.C., & Michos, E.D. (2014). The association of low vitamin D with cardiovascular disease: Getting at the "heart and soul" of the relationship. *Am J Epidemiol, 179*(11), 1288–1290.

Schoenthaler, A., Chaplin, W.F., Allegrante, J.P., Fernandez, S., Diaz Gloster, M., Tobin, J.N., & Ogedegbe, G. (2009). Perception and recall provider communication effects medication adherence in hypertensive African Americans. *Patient Education and Counseling, 75*, 185–191.

Sentry Health Monitors. (2012). *What is blood pressure?* Retrieved June 3, 2012, from http://www.lifeclinic.com/focus/blood/whatisit.asp.

Shadden Laboratory. 2014. Current studies in hypertension and associated risk factors. University of California, Berkeley. Accessed July 22, 2016. https://www.ocf.berkeley.edu/~bpp/wp-content/uploads/2014/03/feb-27-2014-current-studies-in-hypertension-and-associated-risk-factors.pdf.

Shea, M.K., Houston, D.K., Tooze, J.A., Davis, C.C., Johnson, M.A., Hausman, D.B., ... Bauer, D.C. (2011). Correlates and prevalence of insufficient 25-hydroxyvitamin D status in black and white older adults: The health, aging and body composition study. *J Am Geriatr Soc, 59*(7), 1165–1174.

Siddiqi, L., Hoogduin, H., Visser, F., Leiner, T., Mali, W.P., & Blankestijn, P.J. (2014). Inhibition of the renin-angiotensin system affects kidney tissue oxygenation evaluated by magnetic resonance imaging in patients with chronic kidney disease. *J Clinical Hypertension, 16*(3), 214–218.

Sinasac, L. (2012). The community health promotion plan: CKD prevention and management strategy. *Canadian Association of Nephrology Nurses and Technologists, 22*(3), 25–28.

Sine, Richard. 2008. Beyond White Coat Syndrome: Fear of Doctors and Tests can Hinder Preventive Health Care. *WebMD*, accessed July 20, 2016. http://www.webmd.com/anxiety-panic/features/beyond-white-coat-syndrome.

Spence, A.P., & Mason, E.B. (1987). *Human Anatomy and Physiology*. Menlo Park, CA: Benjamin/Cummings.

SPRINT Research Group. 2015. A Randomized Trial of Intensive Versus Standard Blood-Pressure Control. *New England Journal of Medicine*; Nov 26, 373:2103–2116. Accessed July 13, 2016. DOI: 10.1056/NEJMoa1511939.

Stamler, J., Brown, I.J., Yap, I.K.S., Chan, Q., Wijeyesekera, A., Garcia-Perez, I., Chadeau-Hyam, M., ... Elliott, P. (2013). Dietary and urinary metabonomic factors possibly accounting for higher blood pressure of African Americans compared to white Americans: The INTERMAP study. *Hypertension* 62(6): 1074–1080.

Stavropoulou, C. (2011). Perceived information needs and non-adherence: Evidence from Greek patients with hypertension. *Health Expectations, 15*, 187–196. DOI:10.1111/j.1369-7625.2011.00679.x.

Stewart, M. (2013). Qualitative inquiry: Perceptions of sexuality by African Americans experiencing hemodialysis. *J Advanced Nursing*, 69(8), 1704–1713. DOI:10.1111/jan.12028.

Szomba, C. (2012). Understanding obesity and chronic kidney disease. *Nephrology Nursing J*, 39(2), 131–136.

Tamez, H., Kalim, S., & Thadhani, R.I. (2013). Does vitamin D modulate blood pressure? *Curr Opin Nephrol Hypertertension, 22*(2), 204–209.

Tang, L., Xu, T., Li, H., Zhang, M., Wang, A., Tong, W., ... Zhang, Y. (2014). Hypertension, alcohol drinking and stroke incidence: A population-based prospective cohort study among inner Mongolians in China. *J Hypertension, 32*(5), 1091–1096.

Tussing-Humphreys, L., Thomson, J.L., Mayo, T., & Edmond, E.A. (2013). Church-based diet and physical activity intervention for rural, lower Mississippi Delta African American adults: Delta Body and Soul Effectiveness Study, 2010–2011. *Prev Chronic Dis, 10*, 120286. DOI: http://dx.doi.org/10.5888/pcd10.120286.

U.S. Department of Health and Human Services, Office of Disease Prevention and Health Promotion. *Healthy People 2020: About healthy people*. Retrieved November 2, 2014, from http://www.healthypeople.gov/2020/about-Healthy-People.

Uzun, S., Belguzar, K., Mehmet, Y., Filiz, A., Mehmet, B.Y., & Hayrettin, K. (2009). The assessment of adherence of hypertensive individuals to treatment and lifestyle change recommendations. *Anadolu Kardiyol Derg, 9*, 102–109.

Van Horn, L.V., Bausermann, R., Affenito, S., Thompson, D., Striegel-Moore, R., Franko, D., & Albertson, A. (2011). Ethnic differences in food sources of vitamin D in adolescent American girls: The national heart, lung, and blood institute growth and health study. *Nutrition Research, 31*, 579–585.

Venkata, C., Ram, S., Ramaswamy, K., Quian, C., Biskupiak, J., Ryan, A., ... Russo, P.A. (2011). Blood pressure outcomes in patients receiving angiotensin II receptor blockers in primary care: A comparative effectiveness analysis from electronic medical record data. *J Clinical Hypertension, 13*(11), 801–812.

Volpe, M., & Tocci, G. (2013). Olmesartan in the treatment of hypertension in elderly patients: A review of the primary evidence. *Drugs Aging, 30*, 987–998. DOI:10.1007/s40266-013-0130-8.

von Sarnowski, B., Putaala, J., Grittner, U., Gaertner, B., Schminke, U., Curtze, S., ... Tatlisumak, T. (2013). Lifestyle risk factors for ischemic stroke and transient ischemic attack in young adults in the Stroke in Young Fabry Patients study. *Stroke, 44*(1), 119–125. DOI: 10.1161/STROKEAHA.112.665190.

Wang, J., Chen, W., Ruan, L., Toprak, A., Srinibasan, S.R., & Berenson, G.S. (2011). Differential effect of elevated blood pressure on left ventricular geometry types in black and white young adults in a community (from the Bogalusa Heart Study). *American J Cardiology, 107,* 717–722.

Warren-Findlow, J., Seymour, R.B., & Brunner Huber, L.R. (2012). The association between self-efficacy and hypertension self-care activities among African American adults. *J Community Health, 37,* 15–24.

Wedro, B. (2013). *High blood pressure.* Retrieved June 5, 2013, from http://www.emedicine health.com/high_blood_pressure/article_em.htm.

______. (2015). *Kidney Failure: Kidney Failure Facts.* http://www.medicinenet.com/kidney_failure/article.htm.

Weitzman, D., Chodick, G., Shalev, V., Grossman, C., & Grossman, E. (2014). Prevalence and factors associated with resistant hypertension in a large health maintenance organization in Israel. *Hypertension, 64*(3), 501–507. DOI:10.1161/HypertensionAHA.114.03718.

Wexler, R., Feldman, D., Larson, D., Scinnott, L.T., Jones, L.A., & Miner, J. (2008). Adoption of exercise and readiness to change differ between whites and African-Americans with hypertension: A report from the Ohio State University primary care practice–based research network (OSU-PCPBRN). *J Am Board Fam Med, 21*(4), 358–360. DOI:10.3122/jabfm.2008.04.070175.

White, M.F., Kirschner, J., & Hamilton, M.A. (2014). Cardiology patient page: Self-care guide for the heart failure patient. *Circulation, 129,* e293-e294. DOI:10.1161/CIRCULATION-AHA.113.003991.

Whittaker, C., Dunsmore, V., Murphy, F., Rolfe, C., & Trevitt, R. (2012). Long–term care and nursing management of a patient who is the recipient of a renal transplant. *J Renal Care, 38*(4), 233–240.

Wikoff, W.R., Frye, R.F., Zhu, H., Gong, Y., Boyle, S., Churchill, E., ... Kaddurah-Daouk, R. (2013). Pharmacometabolomics reveals racial differences in response to atenolol treatment. *PLoS One, 8*(3), e57639. DOI:10.1371/journal.pone.0057639.

Woo, D., Rosand, J., Kidwell, C., McCauley, J.L., Osborne, J., Brown, M.W., ... Langefeld, C.D. (2013). The Ethnic/Racial Variations of Intracerebral Hemorrhage (ERICH) study protocol. *Stroke, 44*(10), e120-e125. DOI:10.1161/Strokeaha.113.002332.

Woolf, K.J., & Bisognano, J.D. (2011). Nondrug interventions for treatment of hypertension. *J Clinical Hypertension, 13*(11), 829–835.

World Health Organization. (2013). A Global Brief on Hypertension, World Health Day. Accessed July 12, 2016. http://apps.who.int/iris/bitstream/10665/79059/1/WHO_DCO_WHD_2013.2_eng.pdf.

Yamout, H., Lazich, I., & Bakris, G.L. (2014). Blood pressure, hypertension RAAS blockade, and drug therapy in diabetic kidney disease. *Advances in Chronic Kidney Disease, 21*(3), 281–286.

Yan, G., Norris, K.C., Greene, T., Yu, A.J., Ma, J.Z., Yu, W., & Cheung, A.K. (2014). Race/ethnicity, age, and risk of hospital admission and length of stay during the first year of maintenance hemodialysis. *Clin J Amer Soc Nephrology, 9,* 1402–1409.

Zhong, C., Lv, L., Liu, C., Zhao, L., Zhou, M., Sun, W., ... Tong, W. (2014). High homocysteine and blood pressure related to poor outcome of acute ischemia stroke in Chinese population. *PLoS ONE, 9*(9), e107498. DOI:10.1371/journal.pone.0107498.

Zhou, J., Zhang, Y., Arima, H., Zhao, Y., Zhao, H., Zheng, D., ... Yang, J. (2014). Sex differences in clinical characteristics and outcomes after intracerebral hemorrhage: Results from a 12-month prospective stroke registry in Nanjing, China. *BMC Neurology, 14*(172), 1–7.

Index

Numbers in ***bold italics*** refer to pages with illustrations.

access to quality health care 147
account 42
adalat 175
adherence 8; behaviors 116; individual 117; interventions 116; lack of adherence to 116; lifestyle 8, 116; lifestyle regime 116; medication 8
Africa 4
albumin in urine 78
alcohol 17, 18; and stroke 106
Alwall, Nils 89
American Stroke Association 101
angiotensin II receptor blockers (ARBs) 110
anticoagulation therapy 101
appendix 1, 129, 205
arterial blood pressure versus mean arterial pressure 34
Asia 57
atenolol 152
athletes 177
autoimmune kidney disorders 87–88
AV fistula 92

banana 207, 210
Basic Metric Measurement Conversions 205
blister pack ***162***
blood supply 98
blood, urea, nitrogen (BUN) 76; *see also* creatinine
blood vessels ***90***, 149
body mass index (BMI) 50, 79, 81–82; measurement 120
brachial artery 9, ***10***
brain cells 98

calcium 59
Canada 27, 38, 55, 87, 101
Canadian Organ Replacement Register 93
cardiac cycle 9
cardiology 171–172, 174
cardiovascular disease (CVD) 51; cholesterol levels check 191; CVD death rates 52; diabetes 58; mortality risk 71; obesity 189; plaques 58; prevalence 51; risk factors 51, 66, 185, 188–189
catecholamines 202
categories of adherence 122 123; education levels 123; to medicine and lifestyle 123
Centers for Disease and Control and Prevention (CDC) 7, 12, 23, 27, 38
cerebrovascular disease (CVA) 96
Chicago Community Adult Health Study 25
child-bearing age 185
China 55, 101
cholecalciferol therapy 200
cholesterol 47
Christmas 174
chronic kidney disease (CKD) ***74***, 77–79, 85; aging and 80; definition 77, 84; detection 78–79, 85; markers 85; occurrence in women 85; prevalence 77, 80; risk factors 74; stages 85; treatment 80; and weight 80–82
church interventions and Dallas Heart Study 127–128; and Good NEWS trial 127–128
circulation 25 OH vitamin D concentrations 67
classroom 5
clinic visits 38
cohort 4, 71
Colorado Study 44;
complications of vitamin D deficiency 66
control rates 4
coping 173–174
coronary artery disease (CAD) 47, 186; coronary plaque diabetic 61; death rates 56, 94–95; hypercholesterolemia 186; prevalence 58; risk factors 57; risk for rupturing 58, 62; type 2 diabetes mellitus 56–57; women and 190
coronary heart disease (CHD) 47–49; comorbid risk factor in women 190; prevalence 47–49; risk factors 47, 49, 63; and smoking 189
creatinine 76
creatinine-derived eGFR 78
cystatin C blood test 78

databases 4
death 24, 27; obesity 189; premature 53; rates after allograft failure 94–95
dentistry 18, 19
diabetes 47, 57–58, 79
diabetic kidney disease 84; and renin-angiotensin system (RAS) 84; treatment and prevention 84
dialysis 76; definition 8; hemodialysis (HD) 77, 89, ***90***, 173; needle sites ***90***; quality of life 195
dialyzer ***91***
diary 40
diastolic definition 34
diet quality 126
Dietary Approaches to Stop Hypertension (DASH) 117, ***118***, 129, 138
Dietary Guidelines for Americans (DGA) 118–119; and sodium intake restrictions 118
disability-adjusted life year (DALY) 28, 52
disability rates 28
disease 1, 4, 184
distrust 186, 187
DNA 75
doctors 212
Donald 174–175
donor kidneys 86
dual renin-angiotensin system blockade (RASB) 154

echocardiographic risk factors 84
education 123; awareness 110
eGFR 78
electrolyte imbalances 76
end-stage renal disease (ESRD) 25, 57, 75, 77, 79, 80, 86, 88; diabetes and 86; effects 194; ESRD 86; Hispanics 79; kidney transplant 195; patient knowledge 196–197; prevalence 77; transplantation 194; treatment cost 80
England 27, 38
equator 201
Ethnic/Racial Variations of Intracerebral Hemorrhage (ERICH) 10
etiology 5, 20
Europe 77, 83

fiber ***118***
fistula ***90–92***
fruits 117, ***118***, 205

gender 47, 48, 57, 102
genetics 29, 30–31; slavery hypothesis 30
GenSalt Study 121
geometry types 50
Ghent 44
glomerular filtration rate (GFR) 77–78; *see also* eGFR
glycosylation 61
government agencies 185
grains 205
guidelines JNC 8, 11–12

health care practitioner 145
health complications 146
health insurance 147
health records 39
Healthy People 2010 26
Healthy People 2020 Objectives 47, 49
heart **53**
Heart and Stroke Foundation 101; Canada 96
heart disease 47; risk factors 62
heart failure 83; causes **53**; definition **53**; in the elderly 54; pulse risk factors 54; stages 54–55
heart position **35**
Heart 360 web application 42, 43
high plasma Hcy concentration (hHcy) and stroke 105
Hispanics 79
hormone 76
hydrochlorothiazide 172
hypercholesterolemia 109
hypertriglyceridemia 81

injury 186
Ireland 99

Jackson Heart Study 81
Janice 173–174
Japan 4, 11, 87; ABPM cost 46; IgA nephropathy 87–88
Jasper 172–173
JNC 8 Guidelines 153

Kaiser Permanente 41
kidney disease 75–77; aging 77; autoimmune 87–88; causes **74**; diabetes **74**, 77; mutations 75, 94; toxins 76; treatment 76
kidney failure 77, 86; and Hispanics 86
Kidney Foundation of Canada 92
knowledge test 211
Korotkoff's sound 9

labels 119
left ventricular hypertrophy (LVH) 49; and cardiovascular disease 49; defined 49; and geometric patterns 49; pathogenesis 51
LV mass index 155

Medicaid Services 46, 148
medical records 39
medication on the market 150
Medigap supplemental insurance 148
MedSignals pillbox 182–183
memory and cognitive functions 147
metabolics 151
microalbuminuria value 82
mineralocorticoid receptor blockade (MRB) 154
monotherapy 149
morbidity 7, 27, 49, 93
Morisky Medication Adherence Scale MMAS-8 182
mortality 7, 27, 49

multigrain bread 206, 208
"My Chart" 41

National Institute for Health and Care Excellence (NICE) 45
National Kidney Foundation 77, 91–92
nephrons 73
nonpharmacological management 116–117; adherence interventions 122; definition 140; exercise programs 116; lifestyle modifications 117, 122; self-efficacy 138–139; self-management 140

omnivores 201
oxygenation level dependent (BOLD) magnetic resonance imaging (MRI) for kidney imaging 193

patient-physician relationship 147
peritoneal dialysis (PD) 77, 89; *see also* treatment
pharmacological management 145; angiotensin-converting enzyme (ACE) inhibitors 149; angiotensin II inhibitors 149; beta-blockers 149; calcium channel blockers 149; central nervous system agents 149; diuretics 149; medications 149, 150; vasodilators 149
pharmacotherapy 149
phosphorus 59
plasma renin activity 152
policy planners 110, 123, 133, 185
prevention programs 49
proteinuria 37
pulse pressure 191

quality of life 2
Quinton, Wayne 89

reference guide 5
renin 76
renin-angiotensin system (RAS) 150

salt ***118***; consumption 75, 120; hypothesis 30; sodium excretion and income 120 and ventricular mass 29–31, ***118***
screening 181, 204
Scribner, Belding 89
self-care activities 127
self-management 140
self-management of medication 40
serum phosphorus 78
Silastic-Telfon shunt 89; smoking 47, 52, 79
smoking 47, 52, 79
Spain 4
statin 156
stethoscope 10
stress 26, 143–144; stress management 137
stroke 96, 113; avoidance 99–100; belt 101, 108; cause 98; disabilities 98, 99; effects ***104***, 112–113; guidelines 101; life satisfaction after 114–115; lifestyle behaviors 100; lifestyle choices 98–99; mortality 99, 101, 102; prevalence 99, 107; rehabilitation phase 115; risk factors 96–98, 102, 106; signs 103; types 103
systole definition 34
Systolic and diastolic pressures 8–9, 11

target organ 46
technology 39, 40
Thailand 21
Thiazide type 11
Third National and Nutritional Examination Survey 78
toxins 76
transportation 126–127
treatment 77
trials 36, 41
type 2 diabetes 57–58, 79

United States 2, 3, 12, 23, 177, 178, 183, 187, 190
US National Health and Nutritional Examination Survey (NHANES) 154
United States Public Health Service observational syphilis study 187
uric acid 75, 89

vascular auscultation 9
vegetables 117, 205
Visual Analog Scale (VAS) 182
vitamin D 64, 201; deficiency 65, 66, 69, 70; food sources 68; forms 64; function 65; and mortality 69–71; and Rein-angiotensin system (RAAS) 202; risk factors 66, 70; supplements 64, 68, 71
VO_2 max 136

walking impairment questionnaire (WIQ) 129
water 76, 149
white-coat syndrome 19
World Bank 159
World Health Organization 13, 23, 52